Growing up with alcohol

The use and misuse of alcohol by young people is an established concern. Initiatives designed to educate the young about the potential dangers of alcohol are frequently directed solely at teenagers; *Growing up with Alcohol* argues that this may be leaving it much too late.

Emma Fossey presents a detailed account of a study of children aged between five and ten years, carried out through a series of ingenious game-like activities. She explodes the myth that young children are ignorant about alcohol and provides valuable insights into how young children learn about drinking, and about their early perceptions of alcohol. Some of the findings are predictable, some are surprising, others are deeply disturbing. All emphasize the fact that most young people in drinking cultures begin to form their impressions about alcohol at a very tender age. The study questions the effectiveness of past alcohol education and argues strongly that future initiatives should develop innovative and user-friendly alcohol education materials for use in primary schools, as well as in secondary schools and colleges.

Growing up with Alcohol will appeal to a wide range of readers, including social science and psychology students and teachers, researchers and practitioners in alcohol and health education, and policy makers.

Emma Fossey is a Research Fellow in the Alcohol Research Group at the University of Edinburgh.

Growing up with alcohol

Emma Fossey

Foreword by Martin Plant

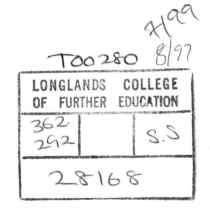
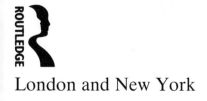

London and New York

First published 1994
by Routledge
11 New Fetter Lane, London EC4P 4EE

Simultaneously published in the USA and Canada
by Routledge
29 West 35th Street, New York, NY 10001

© 1994 Emma Fossey

Typeset in Times by
Florencetype, Kewstoke, Avon

Printed and bound in Great Britain by
Biddles Ltd, Guildford and King's Lynn

British Library Cataloguing in Publication Data
A catalogue record for this book is available from the
British Library.

Library of Congress Cataloging in Publication Data
Fossey, Emma, 1966– .
   Growing up with alcohol / Emma Fossey ; foreword by Martin Plant.
      p.   cm.
   Includes bibliographical references and index.
   1. Children – Alcohol use – Scotland – Edinburgh.   2. Children –
   Alcohol use – England – Birmingham.   I. Title.
   HQ755.8.C354   1994
   362.29′22′083 – dc20   94–8495
                                                                 CIP

ISBN 0–415–09930–7 (hbk)
ISBN 0–415–09929–3 (pbk)

This book is dedicated to my parents,
Arthur and Mary, and to Ken

Contents

List of illustrations

Foreword

Martin Plant

Between birth and the onset of regular drinking behaviour there lies a largely uncharted period of life. Early impressions, social situations and mass media images may set the scene for the later acquisition of patterns of drinking and, perhaps, of negative as well as positive experiences with alcohol. Most adults in industrial societies, as well as many of those in the developing world, consume alcoholic beverages at least occasionally. In many societies the convivial and social use of alcohol is so commonplace and so well entrenched that the invitation to 'have a drink' is synonymous with an offer to join in the imbibing of some form of alcohol. The majority of those who consume alcohol do so in moderation and without serious harm. Even so, the very popularity of alcohol use is such that, perhaps inevitably, some people consume it heavily, inappropriately and with serious, even fatal, results. Such damaging alcohol consumption is perhaps an unavoidable price to pay for having a psychoactive drug that is legal and popular in most parts of the world.

Drinking habits are influenced by a confusing constellation of forces. These include a host of social and environmental factors, as well as the personality, genes and individual life circumstances of each drinker. In societies in which alcohol consumption is legal, at least for adults, public policy generally seeks to foster the harm-free use of alcohol, while attempting to curb alcohol problems and to protect vulnerable groups of people, in particular the young. The latter are widely viewed as being inexperienced and particularly prone to drink in excess and with damaging results. This special concern about the young has prompted a huge amount of activity to educate them, not only about the potential dangers of alcohol, but also about those associated with other risky pleasures.

During the past thirty years per capita alcohol consumption has risen in many countries, though it has also recently generally levelled off or, in some cases, declined. During the period of increasing alcohol consumption most officially recorded rates of alcohol-related problems also increased. At the same time public and political concern has periodically focused on the real or perceived problem of alcoholic excess among the young. Sometimes such concern reflected real events and trends. Sometimes it has served to emphasize the existence of a chronic, but usually ignored phenomenon. Sometimes heightened interest has taken the form of a 'moral panic', by exaggerating and demonizing a problem which is really sufficiently serious not to require amplification.

The reality is that, in all societies in which alcohol is widely used and esteemed, the young by no means have a monopoly of alcohol problems. In fact chronic heavy drinking and 'alcohol dependence' or 'alcoholism' overwhelmingly involve people above the age of twenty-five. The young, in particular adolescents, teenagers and those in their twenties, often drink to intoxication. A substantial proportion experience low-level adverse consequences, such as hangovers and nausea. A minority suffer or inflict more serious harm. This mainly takes the form of accidents, injuries or behaviours that are linked, not to chronic (or daily) heavy drinking, but to periodic heavy consumption.

Because they are perceived as being especially vulnerable and because they are also easy to contact, teenagers have been by far the most frequently selected target for systematic and formal education about alcohol. Teenagers have also been thus targeted because of the belief that they are old enough to be aware of alcohol, yet in many cases to be not quite old enough to be consuming it on a regular basis. It appears to be the case that younger individuals are generally viewed as being too immature either to know or to care much about alcohol, far less to drink it themselves. School students, generally adolescents and teenagers, are a readily accessible captive audience at whom education about alcohol and other social and health issues may be directed. Sadly, health education in many countries is grossly inadequate and is seldom assessed or evaluated. Frequently educational initiatives have relied too heavily on the naive assumption that the provision of factual information will influence behaviours. Those evaluations that have been conducted have generally produced disappointing results about the short-term impact of initiatives. Their longer-term impact is simply unknown. What is clear from the vast literature on alcohol use and its attendant problems is that social and cultural factors exert a considerable influence on drinking habits. The latter frequently change dramatically during an individual's life. The early onset of heavy drinking does not necessarily predict the later development of a chronic 'alcohol problem'. Nevertheless, drinking habits often reflect patterns of alcohol use by parents, peers and significant others. There is little doubt that the family may exert a profound influence on the development of drinking habits or the avoidance of alcohol, just as the family plays a major role in other areas of socialization.

Growing up with Alcohol provides a refreshingly lucid account of one of the few studies to examine the orientations towards alcohol of young children. In so doing, it enters an arena that has daunted most researchers. Such reticence probably reflects a common assumption that children are too difficult to study in this context, or that they are just too young to be of relevance to a behaviour largely linked with the post-adolescent section of the population.

Emma Fossey, a psychologist, set out to replicate and to adapt a classic investigation that had been conducted two decades earlier. The resulting findings from this new study are described in the context of a burgeoning literature about young people and alcohol, and of the difficulties that lie in the way of attempts to reduce the levels of alcohol problems among not only adolescents, but adults too. *Growing up with Alcohol* fills in a large and crucial section of the emerging jigsaw of what we know about how people see alcohol and how their drinking careers may develop. Following in the pioneering footsteps of Professor Gustav Jahoda and Ms Joyce Cramond, this study approached children aged between five and ten years using a battery of ingenious game-like activities. The latter were used, to good effect, to probe and to elucidate how such young subjects view alcohol and its effects upon adults. Some of the results are predictable. Some are surprising. Others are deeply disturbing. All emphasize the fact that most young people in drinking cultures begin to form their impressions about alcohol and its use (or misuse) at a very tender age. Such impressions when they do develop reflect a remarkable degree of gender prejudice. They further make a striking contrast with the fact that, in Britain at least, drinking by adults is neither deviant nor usually harmful and that adolescents have a generally positive view of alcohol.

This study tells the lie to the belief that pre-adolescents neither know nor care about alcohol. They certainly know and many of them also appear to care. Perhaps the latter reflects the fact that, while the early learning experiences of most children involve no major tragedies, some have their young lives ruined by exposure to adult alcohol problems. *Growing up with Alcohol* provides persuasive support for the need to help and equip adults, especially parents, with the information and guidance that may be necessary to inform and guide their children about a substance that most will be consuming regularly by their early to mid teens and for decades thereafter. This study also suggests that there is a need for the development of innovative and user-friendly alcohol education materials for use in primary as well as in secondary schools and colleges. As noted above, in many localities alcohol education is disorganized and is invariably aimed solely at those in secondary (high) schools. Emma Fossey's findings suggest that this may be leaving it much too late.

Martin Plant
Alcohol Research Group
University of Edinburgh
November 1993

Acknowledgements

Before embarking upon this project, I was fortunate to be able to consult with Professors Gustav Jahoda and John Davies, both of whom had been associated with the original study on which the current exercise was based. Many of the original test materials had been preserved, including a film of Joyce Cramond performing the tasks with some children, all of which helped me greatly in the design of my own materials. To this end, I am also extremely grateful to all the children who were involved in the piloting of these new test materials, before the main testing was carried out.

The main fieldwork was made possible only by the cooperation and willing participation of the local Education Authorities, the teachers and the pupils of Edinburgh and Birmingham. I am indebted to all who were involved, for enabling this work to proceed in the enjoyable and smooth manner in which it did, despite the inevitable disruption this must have incurred. To this end I should also like to thank Gill Robinson, Mike Carr and Joe Harvey for overseeing the Birmingham side of the project, and in particular, Erica Coles who conducted the fieldwork in Birmingham so competently.

Throughout the duration of this project, I have received advice and encouragement from colleagues and other friends. Though impossible to mention each by name, my gratitude is extended to all of them. However, special mention must be made of some individuals in particular. The first of these acknowledgements must go to my colleagues, past and present, at the Alcohol Research Group at the University of Edinburgh, in particular Wendy Loretto and Carl May, for their unfailing support and good humour. I am also especially grateful to Anne Pinot de Moira and to Patrick Miller for their seemingly inexhaustible patience in providing statistical advice. The secretaries at the Alcohol Research Group must also be thanked, and in particular Sheila MacLennan for her contribution to the typing of the manuscript, as must Duncan Verrall for his much-appreciated computing skills. Particular thanks also go to Martin Plant, Tom Pitcairn and Ivy Blackburn, my supervisors during this research. I am especially grateful to Martin Plant for his support during the preparation of this book, and for his contribution in the Foreword.

The research project on which this book is based was funded jointly by the Portman Group and the Scotch Whisky Association. Additional support from the Scotch Whisky Assocation made it possible to complete this book.

Finally, special thanks go to my family and to Ken, not only for their prevailing sense of good humour throughout, but also for giving me the vital encouragement, understanding and support which enabled this book to be completed.

Introduction

> a custom, a traditional way of thinking and acting, does not survive and spread from its point of origin unless it gives men some satisfaction, unless it solves some human problem.
>
> (Horton, 1991: 9)

The consumption of alcohol, as a custom, has been with us since ancient times. Its longevity and pervasiveness appear all the more remarkable when one considers the numerous attempts to control or abolish it that have been documented throughout history. Indeed, anthropologists have observed that in the rare cultures in which alcohol use does not exist, the adoption of alternative substances which are perceived to fulfil a similar function has commonly been noted. Examples of these include Jimsonweed, a popular substance in areas such as California and Mexico, and peyote, a drug obtained from the fruit of a cactus plant, which is commonly observed to be used by Native Americans (Horton, 1991). In Britain, however, over 90 per cent of adults currently drink alcohol, at least occasionally. Moreover, as this high figure indicates, the gap between the proportions of male and female drinkers is closing. Although men still make up the greater percentage of consumers, 89 per cent of women are current drinkers (Foster, Wilmot and Dobbs, 1990). In Northern Ireland, too, the number of male drinkers still exceeds that of women, although the overall proportion of abstainers is considerably higher for Northern Ireland than for Great Britain.

More detailed accounts of current trends in alcohol consumption are available elsewhere (e.g. Foster, Wilmot and Dobbs, 1990; Plant and Plant, 1992). Moreover, this book is primarily concerned with tracing the development of alcohol-related knowledge and beliefs in young children, rather than their behaviours in relation to this substance *per se*. However, in order to give an indication of the cultural importance attached to alcohol by British society, and thus to gain a clearer understanding of the prevailing atmosphere in which children are raised, only very brief mention will be made of some of the more relevant trends.

In 1970, around the time of the survey by Jahoda and Cramond (1972) upon which the current project is based, total consumer expenditure on alcoholic beverages in the United Kingdom was £11,552 million. The corresponding figure in 1992 was £15,966 million. These monetary figures are equivalent to constant 1985 prices, in order to demonstrate more clearly the considerable rise in these levels of expenditure. In addition, for the year 1970, the reported amount of absolute alcohol consumed per head of population in the UK was 5.3 litres. This level reached a recent peak in the late 1980s at 7.7 litres. Thus, while the 1992 figure of 7.4 litres remains relatively high, it does reflect an overall downward trend.

As a caveat to the information above, it should be emphasized that these national patterns of alcohol consumption do not imply uniformity in personal use of alcohol. There are numerous variations in individual drinking habits. Men, for example, are more likely to drink, and to drink heavily, than are women; young adults drink more than older adults; and professional adults are more likely than non-professionals to drink alcohol, although the latter are the more likely to drink heavily. Moreover, variations are also apparent on a regional level. Survey data from Foster, Wilmot and Dobbs (1990) have shown that in Great Britain the Greater London region and Scotland as a whole contained the highest proportions of non-drinkers for both males and females. In addition, the greater proportion of male 'heavy' drinkers (defined as consuming 22 units or more per week)* were located in the north and north-west regions of England, while for females the north-west along with the outer south-east region of England contained the highest proportions of 'heavy' drinkers (defined as consuming 15 units or more per week).

Lest these statistics cause alarm, viewed from an international perspective, UK alcohol consumption is relatively low. In comparison with many countries of the world, the United Kingdom remains at an intermediary level. Moreover, within the context of the European Union, only the populations of the Republic of Ireland and Greece drink less, while France remains the highest consumer, at 12.4 litres per head of total population. Even so, the figures go some way to demonstrating just how pervasive is the use of

---

* A unit is equivalent to a public house measure of spirits or to half a pint of normal-strength beer, lager, stout or cider, or to a single glass of wine.

alcohol. It can thus be seen that British children are brought up in a society in which alcohol consumption is an extremely commonplace activity and where abstinence is the preserve of only a minority. Not surprisingly, given this environment, it is with relative ease that children come to learn about alcohol. Moreover, the literature pertaining to young people has indicated that the age at which they are becoming significantly involved with alcohol is decreasing.

It is commonly assumed that the transitional stage from late childhood to early adolescence is the critical period in which the regular use of alcohol begins. To this end, a considerable body of research has focused on alcohol-related issues within this age group, as will become clear in Chapter 2 of this book. The crucial nature of this period is not in question, but recent research has suggested that socialization to alcohol and its use develops from an earlier age (Zucker and Noll, 1987). However, in comparison with the quantity of research carried out on adolescents, relatively few studies have focused on younger age groups. In their classic study entitled *Children and Alcohol*, Jahoda and Cramond (1972) put forward two reasons for this neglect. The first of these stressed the methodological difficulties of testing young children. The second concerned the common and persistent belief that children are 'innocent' with regard to alcohol, and as such would provide a fruitless target for inquiry. A third related concern, which has been raised more recently in connection with the debate regarding alcohol education, is that introducing the topic of alcohol to children at a young age may encourage earlier experimentation with alcohol. The current project aimed to counteract these disclaimers and took as its inspiration the influential work of Jahoda and Cramond (1972). Both their study and my current exercise attempted to trace the development of alcohol-related cognitions in young children.

In the opening chapter of this book, the bases of these objections to the study of young children and alcohol are addressed, followed by a comprehensive review of the existing literature in this area. This is followed, in Chapter 2, by an examination of the survey data relating to youthful patterns of alcohol use, and a critical discussion of subsequent strategies employed to curb youthful misuse of this substance. The remainder of the book describes the present study in full, including the presentation of a detailed description of the methods involved in the testing of young children, together with a full account of the results. In the concluding chapter, the major issues and implications raised by the findings of this project are discussed.

1 The current status of research regarding young children and alcohol

When Jahoda and Cramond (1972) referred to the difficulties associated with testing young children, they were alluding to the fact that previous studies in the general field of alcohol research had tended to rely heavily on the use of questionnaires. Even today, the self-completed questionnaire remains the most widely used investigative tool in this area. However, interpretation of data derived in this way can often be problematic. Not only does it rely, *a priori*, upon subjects' ability to read, but it also relies on the honesty and accuracy of respondents. For example, it has been observed in surveys dealing with the issue of individual levels of alcohol consumption that respondents may often over- or under-report personal consumption levels either unintentionally due to poor memory recall or deliberately in order to present a more 'desirable' picture of themselves (Midanik, 1982a; Duffy and Waterton, 1984; Marsh, Dobbs and White, 1986). A further example of misreporting comes from studies in which subjects are asked the age at which they received their first alcoholic drink. The tendency is for older subjects to report a later age of first drink than younger subjects. It is widely accepted that this trend is an artefact of memory.

The forced-choice questionnaire can often reduce the likelihood that such misreporting will occur. This format consists of predefined finite response categories, which often necessitate a lower level of accuracy, and which may also serve as useful memory prompts for respondents. However, for this same reason, this type of instrument runs the risk of forcing respondents to make a choice they would not otherwise have made (Feldman and Ruble, 1981; Barenboim, cited in Berndt and Heller, 1985). In contrast, while the open-ended questionnaire places no such restrictions on responses, its unstructured format can lead to important information going unreported (Shantz, 1983). A simple illustration of this appears in Jahoda and Cramond's study during which children were asked the following two open-ended questions: *What have you heard people say about these kinds of (alcoholic) drinks?* And, *What have you been told about drunk people?* Sixty-seven per cent of their sample claimed to have heard nothing about alcoholic drinks, the corresponding figure for the second question was 62 per cent, whereas the same children had previously demonstrated via alternative methods that they did in fact possess information relating to these issues.

An alternative method of questioning which does not rely on an ability to read and write, and therefore one which might be more appropriate for children, is the interview. This technique allows the researcher to ask direct and specific questions based on the assumption that respondent and researcher alike share a common level of discourse and understanding of discourse. For communication to be effective it is essential that both the 'transmitter' and the 'receiver' of the message share a similar frame of reference for interpreting the communication. However, while this can often be assumed with relative justification when dealing with adult subjects, the likelihood that two persons will hold a shared frame of reference will be significantly diminished when one of them is a young child:

> For adults, a common level of discourse within a common level of meaning is shared. Although differences in shared meanings exist among adults and lead to communication problems, the probability is that the amount of overlap in consensual meaning between adults is significantly greater than that between adults and children.
>
> (Sigel, 1974: 202)

There are various difficulties specifically associated with the testing of young children, the source of which can invariably be traced back to this fundamental issue of communication. It is also important to stress that this can be a double-edged problem: discrepancies can occur between the researcher's intended question and the child's interpretation of this question; similarly, the researcher's subsequent interpretation of the child's response may not necessarily coincide with the child's intended meaning. Moreover, young children themselves may deliberately structure their responses in order to suit the situation, as they perceive it:

> It is well known that the suggestibility of children makes them very reactive to methodological variations. In all probability, the more

remote the area of inquiry and the more uncertain the child about his/her answers, the greater this reactivity.

(Goodman, 1990: 935)

An interesting study by Goodman (1990) examined children's responses to questions concerning not alcohol but mental retardation, as a function of inquiry method. Goodman's pilot studies indicated that children's responses were highly reactive to the methodology employed. Especially in situations where they were uncertain, children tended to agree with the investigator where possible, opted for a 'yes' answer in preference to a 'no' answer when these were the available options, and tended towards 'ultra-fair-mindedness'. As a result, the same children gave differing responses to questions concerning their perceptions of mental retardation according to the inquiry method. A further example of this comes from Jahoda and Cramond's study of young children's alcohol cognitions. During this investigation, the children referred to the drinking habits of their parents. It became apparent to the authors that the girls in their study group were more likely than the boys to report that only their father drank or that neither of their parents did so. As the authors themselves point out, it is unlikely that such differences in consumption occur between individual families as a result of the sex of the child. Thus one possibility might be that these girls tended to deliberately under-report the level of consumption for the 'sake of appearances'.

While it is apparent that methods of inquiry such as those detailed above are restricted in their usefulness where young children are concerned, greater subtlety can be achieved through the use of experimental procedures. Experiment-based techniques are those in which independent variables, i.e. those factors controlled by the experimenter, are systematically manipulated in order to observe their effects on the subsequent behaviours of the subject – i.e. the dependent variables. Experimental techniques have several advantages in that they facilitate experimenter control over the independent variables and allow for random assignment of subjects to various experimental conditions, both of which provide a more solid basis from which to draw conclusions about cause and effect. Moreover, they can also often be designed in such a way as to obscure the true aim of the test, which has the advantage of lessening the influence of suggestibility on subjects' responses.

Even so, the ability to generalize from data derived from artificial experimental conditions to events encountered in real life settings is also an issue often contested. However, alternative ethological techniques are quite inappropriate in the context of young children and alcohol. The potential for complications arises in ensuring that the variable(s) to be observed in the experimental procedure is/are not being confounded by other intervening variables that remain unrecognized. For example, in their 'Recognition of Smells' task, Jahoda and Cramond were able to acknowledge that children's familiarity with alcohol, as measured by their ability to identify alcoholic odours, may have been obscured by the fact that children were simply poor at identifying odours in general.

Although experiments do not necessarily rely on verbal ability, the verbal commands that invariably accompany the experiment are equally open to misunderstanding. As Adair (1984) observed, for every research study there are potentially two studies: one is that designed by the experimenter; the other is that perceived by the participant. In other words, the interpretation of data derived from experiments relies upon the assumption that the subject's interpretation of the experimental demands of the situation will coincide with that of the experimenter. Again, the likelihood that this assumption will be erroneous will be enhanced when the subject is a young child:

> The child's attention is drawn to something that interests him and he speaks of it. He has some idea that is important to him and he expresses it in whatever form comes most readily to him. He is never required, when he is himself producing language, to go counter to his own preferred reading of the situation – to the way in which he himself spontaneously sees it. But this is no longer necessarily true when he becomes the listener. And it is frequently not true when he is the listener in the formal situation of a psychological experiment.
>
> (Donaldson, 1978: 74)

It is not practicable to discuss with the child his/her interpretation of the experimental demands or the intended meaning of his/her response. Therefore, the experimenter must be sensitive to the child's point of view and ensure that his/her side of the communication is unambiguous. Examples of such disparity between experimental demands and the child's subsequent interpretation of the demands have been ably demonstrated by Donaldson (1978) and her colleagues Hughes and Grieve (in preparation) in their reworkings of several major experiments by Inhelder and Piaget (1964). Piaget was the major pioneer in the field of child development, and even today his work remains extremely influential. However, it has since become apparent that some of his findings have led many to underestimate the rate at which children's cognitive abilities develop. Donaldson and her colleagues subsequently set out to conduct similar experiments to those of Piaget, adopting a format which they believed would be more comprehensible to young children. The performance of their subjects on these modified tasks was considerably better than Piaget's findings would have led one to predict. The reason for this apparent discrepancy, these authors concluded, was that Piaget's perception of the demands of his tasks often had not coincided with his young subjects' perceptions of these same demands.

In summary, for every research technique there are invariably some drawbacks. The task of the researcher is to decide which method will be the most appropriate both to the topic under investigation and to the subjects involved. In the case of young children, studies employing methods which place heavy emphasis on verbal and reading ability will be open to greater misinterpretation. However, recent advances in the fields of developmental and social psychology have made possible the design of more sophisticated and more reliable experimental methods of testing children.

The second of Jahoda and Cramond's explanations concerning children as a neglected study group related to the assumption that children are unconcerned or simply unaware of alcohol and related issues, and as such would constitute a somewhat futile area of inquiry. The studies documented in the following review provide unequivocal evidence to refute this claim. For this reason, further comment on this issue will not be made here.

However, there are two points which need to be raised in connection with the final issue of whether the early introduction of the topic of alcohol will encourage early experimentation. The first concerns the question as it stands. The second relates to the implicit assumption that early experimentation with alcohol is something to be at least frowned upon and at best avoided.

The following literature review will provide evidence showing that children begin to acquire information about alcohol, in whatever form they perceive it to be, from a very early age. Such early learning indicates that children are acquiring this information from within the family environment, well before they encounter any formal introduction to the subject of alcohol. More pertinently, in many cases this awareness extends to children's personal experience of alcohol. Moreover, it does not necessarily follow that children who know about alcohol are more likely to look more positively upon alcohol. Indeed, during these early years children's perspectives on alcohol develop from an initially neutral viewpoint to an increasingly moralistic, pro-abstinence stance.

This leads on to the second point: that it is contestable whether early 'experimentation' with alcohol need always be inappropriate. In several major European countries, socialization to drinking often begins from a very young age. Moreover, there is no indication that these practices are themselves responsible for any greater prevalence of alcohol-related problems. Children in these countries learn how to drink from a very early age, with the emphasis on alcohol not simply as an intoxicant *per se* but as a social enhancer that is secondary to the social occasion itself. The same may also be said to an extent in defence of British customs. However, the normative cultural values and styles of drinking do differ significantly. For example, in the United Kingdom, drinking, especially when it occurs outside the home, is more strongly associated with adulthood and with adult men in particular than seen as a predominantly light-hearted and pleasurable family activity. In addition, the adverse consequences relating to periodic heavy drinking such as intoxication and public disorder as a result of intoxication pose major problems in the United Kingdom. Finally, studies of British adolescent alcohol use and misuse have indicated that those adolescents whose socialization to alcohol occurs primarily within the family environment are less likely than those whose socialization occurs primarily among peers to constitute a group of heavier and more problematic drinkers (Davies and Stacey, 1972; Harford and Spiegler, 1983; Ghodsian and Power, 1987). Thus, the early introduction of children to alcohol can be a positive proposition. Indeed, many researchers and policy makers currently advocate such action.

A REVIEW OF CURRENT LITERATURE ON YOUNG CHILDREN AND ALCOHOL

The first comprehensive attempt to trace the development of young children's knowledge, attitudes and behaviour in relation to alcohol was conducted in Scotland, by Jahoda and Cramond (1972). Two-hundred and forty children between the ages of five and a half and ten and a half participated in the study, which consisted of a series of game-like activities designed to elicit the following aspects of their alcohol cognitions: familiarity with alcohol; attitudes to adult drinking behaviour; awareness of the social norms associated with alcohol consumption; understanding of the concept of alcohol; recognition of the physical manifestations of drunkennes; and, finally, future orientations regarding alcohol. The results of this study were important for two reasons. First, the authors demonstrated that alternative, effective methods of testing children could be developed. Second, they demonstrated that children were aware of alcohol at an early age.

Subsequent to the publication of this report twenty years ago, only a small number of studies have been conducted in this area. The following is a review of the rather limited literature pertaining to young children and their alcohol cognitions. The predominant messages conveyed in all these studies respond to the objections listed above: it is possible to design methodologies that are appropriate for testing young children; children are very much aware of alcohol from an early age; and this awareness, in many cases, extends to children's early personal experience of alcohol.

Children's ability to identify alcohol

Studies that have attempted to obtain objective measures of young children's familiarity with alcohol have commonly used one or other of two techniques. The first of these approaches involves the assessment of children's visual identification of alcoholic beverages, using photographs or unlabelled bottles of various alcoholic beverages; the second, has concentrated on children's ability to identify alcoholic beverages on the basis of odour recognition.

Visual recognition of alcoholic beverages

In a study by Jahoda, Davies and Tagg (1980), 113 children aged between four and seven years were presented with a set of twelve colour photographs of bottles, six of which were of alcoholic drinks (whisky, vodka, wine, sherry, beer, Guinness) and six of which were of non-alcoholic drinks (tomato juice, limeade, lemonade, Coca-Cola, Irn Bru, milk). As part of the study, children were required to 'name' the bottles in each of the photographs. In addition to responses that included the appropriate alcoholic beverage name, any mention of other specific alcoholic drinks or more general descriptions such as 'grown up drinks', were also deemed correct. On this basis, approximately half the children in both the youngest age group (four to five and a half) and the middle age group (five and a half to six and a half) were able to give an appropriate alcoholic-type label to the pictures. In the oldest age group (six and a half to seven and a half), almost two-thirds of the children were successful. Subsequent comparisons between performance on this task and patterns of parental alcohol consumption failed to establish a significant association between the extent of children's knowledge of specific drinks and any aspect of their parents' drinking behaviour.

In the United States, Penrose (1978) reported a similar lack of association between children's ability to identify a series of alcoholic beverages and parental drinking habits. Eighty-nine children aged four and a half to six and a half years were asked to identify a series of alcoholic and non-alcoholic pictures. All the children successfully identified the alcoholic beverage beer, and only 2 per cent failed to identify wine. Not surprisingly, significantly fewer children were able to identify whisky, vodka and tequila. A detailed and more standardized account than that collated by Jahoda, Davies and Tagg (1980) of primarily paternal drinking habits nevertheless failed to distinguish any aspect of paternal drinking behaviour that could significantly be related to the performance of these children.

Both Noll (1983) and Greenberg, Zucker and Noll (1985) also conducted similar studies in the United States, but on groups of younger children. In a small pilot study of seventeen children aged from two and a half to six years, Noll (1983) found that all seventeen were able to identify correctly the photograph of beer. Again, photographs of other alcoholic beverages including wine, gin/vodka, whisky and sherry were less readily identified by the children. Nevertheless, taking all the alcoholic drinks together, the overall success rate for this sample was 52 per cent.

Following on from this pilot study, Greenberg, Zucker and Noll (1985) examined a larger population-based sample of children within the same age range. Within this sample a developmental trend in ability to identify alcoholic beverages was found, with the older children significantly outperforming the younger children. The success rates for these children were 61 per cent and 45 per cent respectively. Differences in cognitive capacity, as measured by the Peabody Picture Vocabulary Test – Revised (Dunn and Dunn, 1981), were not sufficient to explain the developmental trends in identification ability. However, the authors did find a significant relationship between patterns of parental consumption and children's performance. Children whose fathers reported heavy drinking levels displayed a greater knowledge of alcoholic beverage names than children whose fathers reported lighter alcohol consumption. This finding highlights the role of exposure to alcohol in the immediate environment and supports the theory that developmental increases in performance may likewise be due to the increases in exposure to alcohol that inevitably accompany rising age.

The following two studies have examined alcohol identification in samples of slightly older children. Miller, Smith and Goldman (1990) conducted a test of alcohol identification on eighty-nine children aged between six and eleven years. Colour photographs of three alcoholic (beer, wine and liquor) and six non-alcoholic beverages were presented in three rows of three, so that each row contained one picture of an alcoholic beverage. Each child was given a sheet of paper containing an exact replica of one of the rows and his/her task was to circle the picture of 'whisky or beer'. Every child in the sample was able to complete this task successfully. The second study, by Gaines *et al.* (1986), examined children's ability to identify alcoholic beverages using a slightly different technique. Instead of using photographs, the authors presented children with empty and unlabelled bottles of both alcoholic and non-alcoholic beverages. In this study, the younger children (approximately five to six years old) were as successful as the older children (approximately thirteen to fourteen years old). These results, and those of the previous study, imply the existence of a ceiling effect on further age-related increases in identification ability, which occurs roughly around the age of five to six years.

It is important to note that the criteria for successful identification of alcohol differed between these studies. In both Jahoda, Davies and Tagg's study (1980) and that of Penrose (1978), successful identification included any 'alcoholic-type' label, whereas in the other studies children were required to apply the appropriate specific names to the alcoholic drinks. Nevertheless, both types of study demonstrate early developmental trends associated with the ability to recognize and identify alcoholic beverages by sight. In general, knowledge of alcoholic beverage names improved significantly with rising age, up to about six years of age, after which further age increases ceased to significantly enhance performance.

Odour recognition of alcoholic beverages

Children can become familiar with alcohol in a variety of ways, from a number of sources. Such learning processes can be divided fundamentally into two categories: active learning through personal experiences in the immediate environment; and passive learning from sources in the external environment, e.g. the mass media. In many cases, the design of studies is such that it is often difficult to assess accurately which aspects of children's learning are a result of which type of process. It is evident that visual recognition of alcoholic drinks can be the result of either of these learning processes. However, evidence of children's ability to recognize and identify alcohol by smell is strongly indicative of active learning within the home-controlled environment.

In Jahoda and Cramond's study (1972) children's familiarity with alcohol was assessed by means of the 'Recognition of Smells' task. Instead of using photographs or empty bottles, the authors presented children with an array of identical jars, each containing either an alcoholic liquid (beer and whisky) or a non-alcoholic liquid (peppermint, disinfectant, paraffin, soap liquid, perfume, coffee and vinegar). On the initial trial children were asked to say simply whether they recognized each odour. On the second trial, those odours which the children had claimed to recognize were then presented again, and this time children were asked to identify the odours. On the initial trial, 55 per cent of the total sample claimed to recognize the beer odour and 81 per cent claimed to recognize the whisky odour. Following the second trial, the percentage of children who gave an appropriate alcoholic-type label to one or both of the alcoholic odours was as follows: 39 per cent (five and a half to six and a half years); 55 per cent (seven and a half to eight and a half); 61 per cent (nine and a half to ten and a half years). The authors also conducted further tests on nursery-school children and found that of their sample of fourteen four year olds two children were able to identify one or both of the alcoholic odours.

During the main task, it became apparent that a proportion of children were poor at recognizing and identifying odours in general. It is well established that the human capacity for unassisted or 'free' identification of odours is limited (Schab, 1991). Taking this into account, Jahoda and Cramond established an arbitrary cut-off point whereby any children who were unable to identify three or more odours were excluded from analysis. This applied to 68 children in their original sample, the majority of whom belonged to the youngest age group. As a result, the success rates for the remaining sample increased dramatically to 74 per cent, 69 per cent and 71 per cent respectively, and 66 per cent of the nursery children. Furthermore, the age-related differences in success rates for identification now disappeared. The authors tentatively concluded that children are familiar with alcohol from a very early age, and that age-related differences in performance associated with the initial trial of the task could be explained by developmental differences in ability to identify odours generally.

Again, the Michigan State pre-schoolers studies have carried out similar investigations (Noll and Zucker, 1983; Noll, Zucker and Greenberg, 1990). In the latter study, twenty-nine children aged between thirty-one and forty-eight months and twenty-eight children aged between forty-nine and sixty-nine months were presented with three types of odorous substances: 'universal-use' substances, i.e. those used commonly by adults and children (apple juice, Playdoh, popcorn); 'non-controlled adult-use' substances, i.e. those used commonly but not exclusively by adults (coffee, perfume); and 'controlled adult-use' substances, i.e. those used exclusively by adults (beer, wine, whisky, cigarettes). When asked to identify the odours on the initial trial, children were significantly more successful at identification of both the universal-use and non-controlled adult-use substances, than at identification of the controlled adult-use substances. With regard to these latter substances, 57 per cent of the older children gave an appropriate 'alcoholic-type' label to one or more of the three alcoholic odours, while only 21 per cent of the youngest children were able to do this.

In order to counteract the problem encountered by Jahoda and Cramond – i.e. that of confounding familiarity with alcohol with poor ability to name odours – during a second trial the children were also presented with photographs of the substances contained in the smelling jars (Noll, Zucker and Greenberg, 1990). This assisted identification trial resulted in dramatic increases in success rates for all children. Both universal-use and non-controlled adult-use substances continued to be identified significantly more often that the controlled adult-use substances, although this effect was now less robust. The success rates for identification of alcohol also increased, from 57 per cent to 89 per cent for the older children and from 21 per cent to 69 per cent for the youngest children, although the age-related differences in performance remained significant. The finding that age-related differences in ability to identify alcoholic odours persisted within this age group, even when the developmental differences in verbal identification ability had been adjusted for, suggests that some other factor related to age must be responsible. Similarly, the fact that children were significantly more successful at identifying odours that were more familiar to them than alcoholic odours lends further support to the theory that increases in exposure to these odours, opportunities for which will inevitably increase with age, are responsible for the corresponding trends in identification performance within this age group.

In a study by Noll and Zucker (1983) the sample consisted of eighteen children aged between two and a half to six years, from both alcohol-dependent and non-alcohol-dependent families. Those children from alcohol-dependent families showed significantly greater knowledge of alcoholic beverage names on the initial identification trial than did children from non-problematic backgrounds. However, following the second 'assisted identification' trial this difference disappeared. This finding suggests that children from heavier drinking environments have more opportunity to establish and consolidate an association between various alcoholic odours and their verbal labels, due to greater exposure to alcohol. For children in lighter drinking environments, where alcohol is present but less salient, the appropriate verbal label is less likely to be as consolidated and as readily accessible in their memory. Thus, initial ability to identify alcohol is significantly enhanced when parental consumption is heavier, but when verbal identification is assisted, this advantage is diminished.

These studies, dealing with both visual and odour recognition of alcoholic beverages, have demonstrated a clear developmental trend in children's ability to identify alcohol, up to about the age of five to six years. Beyond this age, further rises in age appear to confer little added advantage. There are two possible explanations as to why this might occur. One is that developmental differences in cognitive capacity may account for differences in performance, up to a point at which further cognitive development ceases to confer an advantage in this respect; the other is that as children grow older, they become more familiar with alcohol due to the inevitable corresponding increase in opportunities for exposure to alcohol, and this continues to affect performance until a ceiling point is reached. This latter explanation appears to be more consistent with the present evidence, at least in relation to the particular age groups studied.

Children's understanding of the concept of alcohol

As noted in the previous section, it is apparent that young children are familiar with alcohol to the extent that they can identify various alcoholic drinks by sight and by smell. For the younger children, identification may be as simple as knowing that alcoholic drinks are 'grown up drinks', whereas older children are more likely to know specific names of alcoholic beverages. However, the ability to identify alcohol does not necessarily imply that children understand the concept of alcohol as a distinct and logical class of drinks.

This has been demonstrated in the study by Jahoda, Davies and Tagg (1980). As mentioned previously, Jahoda and his colleagues tested a group of 113 children aged between four and seven years. They found that for the younger children (aged four and a half to six and a half years), ability to label pictures of alcoholic beverages was not an indicator of ability to explain alcoholic/non-alcoholic groupings – i.e. although roughly half of these children could name the bottles in the pictures and roughly half were able to explain the groupings on the basis of an alcoholic/non-alcoholic division, the same children were not necessarily able to do both. On the other hand, with the older children (aged six and a half to seven and a half years), there was a significant relationship between the number of children (i.e. roughly two-thirds of the group) who were able to name the bottles and the number who were able to explain the groupings.

In the pioneering study by Jahoda and Cramond (1972), the authors also designed a task which attempted to examine the age at which children acquire an understanding of the concept of alcohol. In this experiment, children were presented with a selection of bottles of alcoholic drinks (wine, sherry, whisky and beer) and non-alcoholic drinks (milk, lemonade, Coca-Cola and orange juice), placed at random on a table in front of them. The task required children to separate the eight bottles into two groups of four, so that one group contained bottles that were similar to each other in some way but different to the bottles in the other group. The children were then asked to explain the difference between their two groups. The correct response was to group the bottles according to the alcohol/non-alcohol division. If the children did not group the bottles in this way, the experimenter regrouped the bottles accordingly and the child was given another opportunity to explain this subsequent regrouping. Only 42 per cent of the youngest children performed the initial stage of this task correctly, with 40 per cent then giving the correct explanation. However, following the experimenter's regrouping, a further 26 per cent were able to provide the correct explanation, giving a total of 66 per cent for this youngest age group. The older children were considerably more successful. Ninety per cent of the eight year olds and 96 per cent of the ten year olds successfully performed the alcohol grouping, with all but one child in each age group able to provide the correct explanation. Following the experimenter's regrouping, a further 6 per cent and 3 per cent respectively went on to give the correct response, giving respective totals of 95 per cent and 98 per cent for each age group. The phrasing of children's explanations of bottle groupings also varied significantly with the age of the children. Not one of the youngest children mentioned the term 'alcohol'. In fact, only 11 per cent of the total sample applied this term to the groupings, most of whom belonged to the oldest age group. The most popular way of expressing the groupings, irrespective of age, was to give the name of specific alcoholic drinks.

It is important to note that prior to this task, the children received a training task which followed a similar procedure using fruit and non-fruit items, in order to orientate them to the demands of the main task. Ninety-two per cent of the sample were able to discriminate accurately between these two categories of foods, with almost the same numbers able to provide an accurate verbal description. In comparison, 74.5 per cent of the total sample were able to perform the alcohol groupings correctly, and a further 11.75 per cent were able to give the appropriate explanation following the experimenter's regrouping, giving a total of just over 86 per cent.

It would appear, then, that although many children are able to recognize and identify alcoholic beverages at an early age, most do not possess an operational concept of alcohol until about the age of seven or eight years, at roughly the same time as verbal concepts of more salient groups, e.g. fruit, are being developed. However, the acquisition of a verbal concept of alcohol appears to develop at a later stage, probably around the age of ten years.

Children's awareness of socio-cultural norms relating to use of alcohol

Over the past thirty years total alcohol consumption in the UK has undergone a number of changes. In 1979, consumption peaked at approximately 8 litres of absolute alcohol per head of population. This was followed by a marked decline, although currently consumption is once again on the increase. Today, over 90 per cent of British adults drink alcohol at least occasionally. Young people drink more than older people; males drink more often and more heavily than females (Goddard and Ikin, 1988). Females also generally experience fewer alcohol-related problems than do men (Plant, 1990). However, there is now a tendency for more British women (89 per cent) to consume alcohol, if only in small amounts (Foster, Wilmot and Dobbs, 1990). A number of studies have investigated the extent of children's awareness of cultural norms such as these, in relation to drinking alcohol.

Jahoda and Cramond (1972) investigated children's perceptions of the likes and dislikes of three social groups – i.e. men, women and children – in relation to alcohol-related behaviours. Children listened to audio-taped lists of alcohol- and non-alcohol-related activities, and were asked to indicate how much they thought men, women and children liked or disliked these activities. The alcoholic activities consisted of drinking beer, drinking whisky, going to a public bar and being drunk. The non-alcohol-related activities included items such as mending a car, sewing on buttons and drinking milk. Also included in these lists were several tobacco-related items, i.e. smoking a cigarette and smoking a pipe. The results showed that men were consistently perceived as enjoying alcohol-related activities, with the exception of 'being drunk'. Women were invariably perceived as disliking these activities, often to the same extent as children themselves. The degree of perceived liking for men tended to decrease with rising age of the subjects, although this did not always reach statistical significance with every alcohol-related item.

The difficulty with this particular test is that it is unclear whether children were basing their observations on men and women in general, or more specifically on their parents. It has been suggested that younger children tend to refer to their parents when asked to rate adult preferences, whereas older children are more likely to refer to popular media figures (Higgins, Feldman and Ruble, 1980). This is especially pertinent to Jahoda and Cramond's task in which children were asked to use as a term of reference '*a man/woman – somebody like your father/mother*'. However, these researchers attempted to test this theory by comparing the perceptions of children from abstinent backgrounds with the perceptions of children from heavy drinking backgrounds. The results suggested that children were basing their responses primarily upon their domestic experiences. However, two points should be noted: during the study there were no specific questions concerning parental habits, so the categorizations are based solely on spontaneous remarks made by the children; similarly, the number of children who did make such remarks is relatively small (nineteen claimed their parents were 'abstainers', while eighteen reported 'heavy' drinking parents).

In the study by Jahoda, Davies and Tagg (1980) this younger sample of children was shown drawings of, in turn, a man, a woman, a boy and a girl engaged in the act of drinking something from a glass. They were then asked to choose from six photographs of non-alcoholic drinks and six of alcoholic drinks, three drinks that the person in the drawing would most like to be drinking. Over a third of the youngest children (four and a half to five and a half years) were able to accurately discriminate between adult and child drinks on this basis. Predictably, the number of accurate discriminations rose as age of subject increased. No significant relationship was found between children's perceptions of social drinking norms and parental drinking habits.

Similar studies of children's awareness of cultural norms have also been carried out in the United States. Spiegler (1983) replicated Jahoda and Cramond's 'Perceived Likes/Dislikes' task on a sample of sixty children, also aged between six and ten years. Her sample displayed similar patterns of perceptions to that of Jahoda and Cramond, with greater liking attributed to men and greater dislike attributed to women and children. The 'Appropriate Beverage' task by Penrose (1978) was also designed to examine children's awareness of drinking norms. This author presented a sample of five- and six-year-old children with a series of drawings of festive occasions (e.g. a Thanksgiving dinner, a Fourth of July picnic, a New Year's Eve party and a birthday party) and non-festive events (e.g. watching television, having lunch) in which various male or female, adult or child figures appeared. Five pictures of alcoholic beverages (beer, wine, whisky, vodka and tequila) and five of non-alcoholic beverages (milk, coffee, lemonade, Coca-Cola and orange juice) were also presented. Children were then required to guess which of the drinks the people in the pictures would like to drink, by pointing to, touching or naming one of the beverage photographs. The results showed that children were not only able to discriminate between adult- and child-appropriate drinks, but were also able to discriminate between alcoholic drinks appropriate for festive occasions and non-alcoholic drinks for non-festive occasions. These subjects also chose more alcoholic drinks for adult males than for adult females over all occasions. However, like Jahoda, Davies and Tagg (1980), Penrose found no relationship between children's awareness of these social norms and parental drinking practices.

Greenberg, Zucker and Noll (1985), also used the 'Appropriate Beverage' task on their sample of two-and-a-half to six-year-old children. These authors found developmental differences in relation to awareness of socio-cultural norms, with the older children displaying greater consolidation than younger children, of the norms that adults drink alcohol and children do not, and that men drink more than women. Furthermore, the authors found that children whose fathers reported drinking for escape-related motives tended to perceive greater levels of alcohol consumption among adults than children whose fathers did not. Finally, Greenberg and his colleagues (1985) also examined performance on this task in relation to parental race. As might be expected in a test of cultural norms, there were differences in performance according to race. Both Caucasian and

African-American children selected fewer alcoholic drinks as drinking choices than did children of other races, such as the Hispanic subjects.

The results of these studies indicate that children as young as two and a half show some awareness of normative drinking habits. Developmental differences in awareness of various socio-cultural norms appear up to around the age of five years, at which point these basic norms appear to become consolidated in the minds of children. The question of parental influence remains to be clarified, although the current evidence indicates that more extreme patterns of parental alcohol consumption may exert some degree of influence on children's perceptions of normative drinking behaviour.

Children's alcohol expectancies

So far, little has been mentioned in relation to children's knowledge of alcohol *per se*. The following section describes a number of studies which have investigated various aspects of children's knowledge of alcohol.

In addition to the main battery of tests, Jahoda and Cramond asked their sample a number of informal questions. One of these dealt with the kind of general information children had heard regarding alcoholic drinks. The majority of children (67 per cent) could not recall having heard anything about the drinks, although this finding is probably due to the imprecise nature of the question. Of the seventy-nine children who did report some item of information, just over 73 per cent, the significant majority, who were from middle-class backgrounds, mentioned knowing something negative about alcohol. Moreover, the principle source of this information was the parents.

In a similar vein, Casswell *et al.* (1983) asked their sample of New Zealand nine year olds: *What do you know about what happens to people who drink beer, whisky, wine or any other alcoholic drinks?* The majority of responses referred to acute adverse effects of alcohol consumption, with 71 per cent of the children mentioning drunkenness and only one-fifth of these adding the qualification that amount of alcohol consumed would be a prerequisite factor. Fifteen per cent mentioned more long-term adverse consequences, and only 9 per cent mentioned effects that were associated with more positive aspects of alcohol. On this occasion, the children cited the television as the primary source of their knowledge (35 per cent), with parents (26 per cent) and other miscellaneous sources (24 per cent) following respectively.

More rigorous examination of children's perceptions of the effects of alcohol and adult motives for drinking has been conducted by Gaines *et al*. (1988). Gaines and his colleagues tested eighty children aged from five to thirteen years, by means of six short vignettes depicting one of three drinking situations: escape from painful affect; facilitation of social interaction; and celebration of a positive event. Each child received one of the six vignettes in which the protagonist was either a man or a woman. After hearing the vignette, children were asked a series of questions concerning their understanding of the protagonist's motives for drinking. The highest possible score was given to responses that contained a coordinated psychological antecedent and consequence – e.g. she was feeling nervous and the drink calmed her down. The youngest children (those of five years) were the least successful on this task. Children in the next age group (those aged eight years) performed significantly better than the former group, but also had significantly lower scores than children in the two older age groups (eleven years and thirteen years). Almost 75 per cent of the oldest children could provide coordinated responses. Scores for all children were lowest when the vignette dealt with social anxiety. In addition, girls generally achieved higher scores than boys. In relation to parental drinking, which was quantified by the number of days per year that drinking had occurred in the child's presence, a significant relationship with understanding of adult motives for drinking was found only with the eight-year-old children.

More recently, Miller, Smith and Goldman (1990) examined the development of alcohol expectancies in young children, aged from six to eleven years. Their procedure for assessing children's alcohol-related expectancies (CARE) was partly based on the Alcohol Expectancy Questionnaire – Adolescent (AEQ–A), designed by Christiansen, Goldman and Inn (1982), and consisting of a list of possible consequences of consumption. Male and female hand-puppets were used to represent male and female drinkers. It was found that children's alcohol expectancies became more positive with rising age, with the largest increase occurring with the eight- to nine-year-old children. There were no differences according to gender of the child or gender of the drinker. However, children of fathers who reported no family history of alcohol problems tended to express more positive alcohol expectancies than children with a family history of alcohol dependence.

It is difficult to draw general conclusions about children's knowledge of alcohol from these studies as the nature of the questions differed from study to study. It would appear that the negative short-term consequences of alcohol consumption are more salient to young children. However, this does not necessarily imply that they do not possess a more complex understanding of the issue, as demonstrated by Gaines *et al.* (1988). Generally, as children grow older, i.e. between eight and eleven years, a more mature understanding of adult drinking motives develops, and more positive expectancies about alcohol are reported. Again, it appears that children whose family history suggests more extreme patterns of alcohol involvement are more likely to give responses that reflect these patterns.

Children's ability to recognize drunkenness

The preceding section revealed that children are very much aware of drunkenness as a major consequence of drinking alcohol. However, familiarity with this term does not necessarily imply a thorough knowledge of the physical implications of intoxication. In order to test children's ability to recognize the physical manifestations of drunkenness, Jahoda and Cramond (1972) devised a silent film containing the following sequences: (a) a man in a public bar drinking whisky and then picking up a glass of beer; (b) the man draining the beer glass and staggering from the bar; (c) the man staggering out of the bar door; and (d) the man staggering along the road. Children were shown the film in reverse chronological order, cumulatively, i.e. part d was followed by parts cd, parts bcd, and finally the complete film was shown. Following the first part of the film presentation, i.e. part d, only fourteen children (5.8 per cent) failed to realize that the man was drunk, the majority of whom were from the youngest age group. By the third presentation, i.e. parts bcd, all the children had successfully recognized the man to be drunk. Finally, when children were asked where they had seen people like that before, 95 per cent said they had seen a drunk person first hand.

In response to the high success rates of their main sample, Jahoda and Cramond conducted a similar test on a sample of fourteen four-year-old nursery-school children. Three of these children recognized the physical signs of drunkenness after part d, and only two failed to do so following the presentation of the entire film. No other studies have dealt with this issue, but it is apparent that children learn to recognize the physical manifestations of drunkenness, often through live encounters, from an early age.

Children's attitudes to drinking alcohol

The development of attitudes towards adult drinking behaviour is another aspect of children's early alcohol cognitions that has been the focus of several studies. In their study, Jahoda and Cramond (1972) designed the 'Judgement of Photographs' task to measure children's attitudes towards adult drinking behaviour. A series of photographs of individual men and women engaged in either an alcohol-related activity (drinking beer or whisky) or non-alcohol-related activity (e.g. playing cards, drinking milk, reading a newspaper) was presented to the children. Children then placed each photograph into a response box with four compartments labelled 'Like very much', 'Like a little', 'Do not like a little', 'Do not like very much'. The five to six year olds in this sample reported relatively neutral attitudes towards male adult drinkers, but attitudes to female drinkers already displayed a fairly negative nature at this stage. As age of subject increased, attitudes to drinkers of both sexes became more negative. However, at all ages, children were more condemnatory of female drinkers than of male drinkers.

Using the 'Judgement of Photographs' technique with a sample of sixty children, Spiegler (1983) found that although the attitudes to drinking of her young US sample were also generally negative, they did not differ with respect to the gender of the drinker. She did, however, find similar but less clear-cut age-related trends, with the older children displaying more negative attitudes than the youngest children. However, the eight-year-old children displayed more positive attitudes to both male and female drinkers than any other age group. This was principally due to the positive attitudes towards male and female drinkers of the boys within this age group. It is perhaps important to note that Spiegler's sample was subdivided into five distinct age groups – i.e. five years, six years, seven years, and so on, with each age group consisting of five girls and five boys, as opposed to Jahoda and Cramond's larger and broader age groups. Thus the positive attitude of the eight-year-old age group as a whole is primarily based upon the attitudes of only five boys, and as such should be interpreted with caution.

Finally, using the 'Judgement of Photographs' task in a study conducted in New Zealand, Casswell *et al.* (1985) reported distinctly negative attitudes towards adult drinkers in their sample of 743 eight- to nine-year-old children. Once again, a more pronounced negative attitude was displayed towards the female drinkers. Small, but nevertheless significant, relationships were found between the child's own frequency of consumption and parents' drinking frequency and daily levels of consumption. More intense negative attitudes were displayed by children who reported themselves to be minimal drinkers or abstainers. On the other hand, more positive attitudes were reported by children whose parents reported both greater frequency of drinking and greater daily amounts consumed. Lastly, those children whom parents believed to be more aware of alcohol problems in their environment also tended to hold more negative attitudes. However, of further significance is the finding that, within this latter group of children, there was no significant association between their more negative attitudes and their parents' consumption of alcohol.

These studies indicate that although children may acquire knowledge relating to alcohol and its use at an early age, the development of attitudes towards drinking is slightly slower to occur. The finding that children may be more condemnatory of female drinkers than of male drinkers coincides with the findings of studies examining perceptions of normative drinking patterns, in which women are judged by children to dislike drinking alcohol, often to an extent similar to themselves. In relation to parental influence, the theory that more extreme drinking habits may have more influence on children is again supported. Furthermore, it is interesting to note that when other more pertinent issues are present, e.g. alcohol problems in the immediate social environment, these more salient factors assume greater importance.

Children's self-reported experience of alcohol

In the previous sections, the extent of children's knowledge of various aspects of alcohol has been discussed. This section deals with children's personal experience of alcohol. This is followed finally by a discussion of children's future intentions regarding alcohol.

This particular aspect of children's familiarity with alcohol was also investigated by Jahoda and Cramond (1972). A total of 60 per cent of their sample claimed to have tasted one or more types of alcoholic drink. Moreover, boys were significantly more likely than girls to have tasted alcohol. While the younger children tended to mention more drinks of low alcoholic content than did the older children, this did not reach statistical significance. Finally, approximately 85 per cent of those who claimed to have tasted an alcoholic drink said that their father had provided the taste.

In their study of 743 nine-year-old children, Casswell *et al.* (1983)

noted that 93 per cent of all children in this sample claimed to have had at least a sip of alcohol. This high figure was confirmed by the fact that only 8 per cent of the mothers of these children reported that their children had never tasted of alcohol. The modal age reported by the children for their first taste was seven years, although roughly two-thirds of the mothers estimated this age to be five years or younger. In accordance with the findings of Jahoda and Cramond (1972), the father was identified as the provider of the drink by the majority of the children.

The age at which most people recall having received their first alcoholic drink is commonly reported to be around twelve years. However, it is also widely held that the occasion of the first taste or sip of alcohol probably occurs at an earlier age. The results of these studies provides further confirmation of this. The findings that boys are more likely than girls to have tasted alcohol, and that the father is commonly the provider of the first drink, are also supported by evidence from studies which have examined these issues in relation to older children (Davies and Stacey, 1972; Aitken, 1978; Plant, Peck and Samuel, 1985; Bagnall, 1988).

Children's future intentions regarding alcohol

Finally, Jahoda and Cramond (1972) point to clear age-related differences in the responses of their sample to the question: *Do you think you will drink these (alcoholic drinks) when you are older?* The majority of five to six year olds replied positively (70 per cent), while 25 per cent replied that they would not. In the middle age group the most frequent response was still 'yes' (56 per cent), while 38 per cent now said 'no'. However, in the nine- to ten-year-old group, the majority (48 per cent) now said 'no' to this question and only 41 per cent said that they would drink.

The finding that as children grow older they are less likely to report a positive intention to drink in the future is nicely illustrated by the three studies that have investigated this issue. The study by Noll and Zucker (1983) included children whose mean age was four and a half years. Of this sample, 90 per cent claimed that they would drink when they grew older. The mean age of Jahoda and Cramond's study group was eight and a half years, and of this sample, 56 per cent of these children responded positively. Finally, the mean age of Gaines *et al.*'s sample (1986; 1988) was ten years. Approximately 41 per cent of these children replied affirmatively or at least conditionally affirmatively. This common tendency for many young children to deny the intention to drink in the future should not be considered a reliable predictor of actual behaviour. For, as the following chapter will show, the vast majority of young people do grow up to become drinkers.

2 Trends in youthful alcohol consumption and existing strategies in alcohol education

The collection of data associated with the drinking habits of young people is a relatively recent exercise. The predominant method by which this has been accomplished has consisted of self-report questionnaire surveys and interviews. However, there are two fundamental problems to be borne in mind when interpreting such data: the first concerns sample bias relating to non-responders; the second relates to the question of accuracy in the self-reports of those who do respond (Skog, 1991). With regard to the first of these concerns, it is widely held that drug users who exhibit heavier patterns of use are more likely to be non-respondents (Hauge and Nordlie, 1983). On the other hand, it has been shown that those who do respond often under-report the extent of their drug use:

> Respondents often report drinking less than they actually do, either because they forget, or, particularly among adolescents because they feel it prudent to deny drinking. It is also possible that some adolescents will be subject to poor recall, particularly when drinking occurred in informal circumstances and was not properly measured on licensed premises.
>
> (Marsh, Dobbs and White, 1986: ix)

This trend has been confirmed by studies in which official sales figures for alcohol have typically been found to be considerably higher than quantity estimates of alcohol use (Pernanen, 1974; Midanik, 1982a; Duffy and Waterton, 1984). In a study by Plant, Peck and Samuel (1985), Plant and his colleagues conducted a follow-up survey of young people, in which several questions relating to subjects' experiences of alcohol and other drugs which had been present in their original survey were then repeated. A number of discrepancies became apparent between subjects' initial responses and those recorded on the second occasion of testing. While a propensity for misreporting was likely to account for some of these inconsistencies, it was unclear whether this was due to the incidence of over-reporting at the time of initial testing, and/or the incidence of under-reporting following the second data collection. However, evidence from other research suggests that the tendency for respondents to report false positives, i.e. to claim to have used drugs when they have not, (Single, Kandel and Johnson, 1975; Barnea, Rahav and Teichman, 1987) or to over-report consumption levels (Midanik, 1982b), occurs less frequently.

Although it is not always possible to ensure against incidents of misreporting in survey data, methodological problems such as these are commonly acknowledged in the literature. Moreover, the likelihood of their occurrence is often taken into account by researchers, in terms of both the design of studies and subsequent analyses of the data. With respect to study design, comparisons between daily drinking diaries, quantity–frequency measures and retrospective drinking diaries have commonly shown that the former tend to yield more accurate reports of both drinking frequency (Sobell *et al.*, 1989) and duration of drinking event (Samo, Tucker and Vuchinich, 1989). Furthermore, higher consumption levels have also been reported using this method (Lemmens, Knibbe and Tan, 1988; Corti *et al.*, 1990), confirming the theory that alternative questionnaire methods do tend to produce underestimations of adolescent alcohol consumption. In relation to similar problems at the stage of data analysis, Marsh, Dobbs and White (1986: 31) excluded from analysis a number of questionnaires, typically of young males, in which respondents 'claimed to be drinking sufficient alcohol in a week to prove fatal to creatures larger than themselves'. Similarly, Plant and Foster (1991) excluded all self-reports of consumption levels on the last drinking occasion that were in excess of 32 units of alcohol, i.e. equivalent to drinking 16 pints or more of normal strength beer, lager or cider.

In spite of such difficulties, surveys of this kind have provided valuable insight into the nature of the phenomenon of youthful drinking, from both a regional and a national perspective. Furthermore, these studies have examined a wide range of factors relating to adolescent alcohol use, ranging in scope from young people's earliest experiences of alcohol, through to the experimental drinking stage, and finally to the acquisition of stable drinking patterns. The following review is set out according to this chronological sequence, representing the processes by which adolescents acquire initial experience of alcohol and eventually establish drinking patterns. The first section relates to the initiation stage whereby young people gain personal experience of alcohol for the first time. The second section describes the development and establishment of drinking patterns adopted by adolescents as they become involved in the process of socialization into adulthood. The final section deals specifically with those young people whose drinking habits give cause for concern. This includes so-called 'heavy drinkers' and drinkers who experience alcohol-related problems as a result of their consumption. Finally, these national data are then set in the wider context of international trends in youthful alcohol consumption.

ADOLESCENT DRINKING

Early experiences with alcohol

Most people receive their first real drink of alcohol when they are still quite young. This commonly occurs around the age of eleven to twelve years (Hawker, 1978; Plant, Peck and Samuel, 1985; Marsh, Dobbs and White, 1986; Bagnall, 1988; Plant *et al.*, 1990). On average, boys tend to receive their first drink approximately one year earlier than girls (Hawker, 1978; Plant, Peck and Samuel, 1985). Even so, it is worth noting that both boys and girls often experience their first taste of alcohol – commonly in the form of a sip from their parents' drinks – at a slightly younger age (Marsh, Dobbs and White, 1986; Bagnall, 1988).

So prevalent is this phenomenon, that the proportion of adolescents who, when surveyed, claim never to have personally experienced alcohol is consistently very low. For example, in a study of 1,036 fifteen to sixteen year olds conducted in the Lothian region of Scotland (Plant, Peck and Samuel, 1985), the proportion of both males and females who had never tasted alcohol was only 2 per cent. Likewise, a more recent study of English teenagers, revealed that only 4 per cent of fifteen to sixteen year olds claimed never to have tasted alcohol (Plant *et al.*, 1990). Finally, in a survey conducted in three areas of Britain (Berkshire, England; the Highland region of Scotland; and Dyfed, Wales) a similar percentage of thirteen year olds who had never received a taste of alcohol was reported by Bagnall (1988).

The provider of these first alcoholic drinks is commonly reported to be one or both parents, and invariably such events occur in the home setting (Hawker, 1978; Plant, Peck and Samuel, 1985; Bagnall, 1988). However, a study by Aitken (1978) concerning parental attitudes towards drinking among young people provided somewhat paradoxical results in light of these findings. Forty-six per cent of the adults surveyed stated the belief that children under the age of eighteen years should not be allowed to taste alcoholic drinks. In addition, 63 per cent also felt that children below the age of eighteen should not be allowed to consume small alcoholic drinks at home with their parents.

Why this double standard should occur is unclear. It should be emphasized that in the United Kingdom it is legal for children of five or more years to consume alcohol. Moreover, available evidence indicates that children who drink in the absence of their parents tend to drink more than those whose drinking occurs under parental supervision (Aitken, 1978). It has also been suggested that excessively restrictive sanctions on drinking imposed by parents can foster clandestine drinking among young people (Davies and Stacey, 1972; McKechnie *et al.*, 1977). Findings such as these have led many campaigners to advocate the demystification of alcohol by its early introduction to children in the home. Indeed, in a recent consultation report by the Home Office, the question of the possible introduction in England and Wales, of licensed 'café-style' premises has been raised. When accompanied by an adult, children under the age of fourteen years would be legally permitted to remain on such premises until 8 p.m. in the evening:

> The benefits could be . . . To facilitate the provision of premises where sensible drinking in a mixed, family environment is the norm, instead of the heavy, binge drinking, by groups of young men, which can culminate in alcohol-related disorder.
>
> (Home Office, March 1993: para. 3.3)

Patterns of consumption among young people

The majority of young people in Britain drink alcohol, if only infrequently. The survey literature indicates that in most samples, the proportion of adolescent non-drinkers falls consistently below 10 per cent (Goddard and Ikin, 1988; Sharp, Greer and Lowe, 1988; Foster, Wilmot and Dobbs, 1990; Goddard, 1991; Plant and Foster, 1991). On most occasions where drinking does occur, the amount of alcohol involved is typically small (Bagnall, 1988). Although data relating specifically to adolescents in Ireland (O'Connor, 1976) and Northern Ireland (Loretto, 1993a), suggests that these early experiences are more likely to occur outside of the home, in Britain such activities during the early teenage years are more commonly confined to the parental home.

As a group, boys generally report higher weekly consumption levels and higher levels of consumption on last drinking occasion than do girls (Plant, Peck and Samuel, 1985; Plant *et al.*, 1990; Plant and Foster, 1991). Consumption rates increase for both boys and girls as they become older, and are accompanied by a growing tendency to drink outside of the family setting. Girls tend to reach 'adult' levels of consumption and drinking frequency at around sixteen to eighteen years, at which point these patterns become stabilized (Plant, Peck and Samuel, 1985; Health Education Authority, 1989, 1990; Foster, Wilmot and Dobbs, 1990). For boys, the increase in consumption and frequency is sharper and more prolonged, and can exceed normative 'adult' levels (Plant, Peck and Stuart, 1982). However, for the majority of both males and females, these levels of consumption generally remain within the 'low-risk levels' identified by the Royal College of Psychiatrists (Plant, Peck and Samuel, 1985; Marsh, Dobbs and White, 1986; Goddard and Ikin, 1988; Health Education Authority, 1989, 1990; Plant and Foster, 1991).

Nevertheless, there is a substantial minority of young people whose self-reported consumption levels have been defined as 'heavy', by researchers. In a study of fourteen to sixteen year olds in England, Plant *et al.* (1990) found that of the younger age group (fourteen years), 5.4 per cent of males and 7.1 per cent of females were heavy drinkers. These proportions increased with age, with 13.5 per cent of sixteen-year-old males and 15.5 per cent of sixteen-year-old females reporting consumption rates that would classify them as heavy drinkers. In their Scottish sample, Plant and Foster (1991) found a similar age-related increase in the proportion of heavy-drinking adolescents, although the overall proportion of heavy drinkers was significantly greater for these Scottish teenagers than for their English counterparts. Broadly similar national differences were also noted by Marsh, Dobbs and White (1986). However, it should be pointed out that the criteria for defining 'heavy drinking' often differs between studies. Of those studies which have defined heavy drinking in males as being the equivalent to drinking 50 or more units per week (Plant, Peck and Samuel, 1985; Marsh, Dobbs and White, 1986; Goddard and Ikin, 1988; Goddard, 1991), the proportion of heavy drinkers falls consistently below 5 per cent. Similarly, in studies in which the lower threshold of female heavy drinking is commonly defined as being between 31–36 units per week, the proportion of females drinking at these levels also tends to remain below 5 per cent (Plant, Peck and Samuel, 1985; Goddard and Ikin, 1988; Foster, Wilmot and Dobbs, 1990; Goddard, 1991).

Several studies have also attempted to assess whether such heavy drinking patterns during early teenage years are predictive of future use (Plant, Peck and Samuel, 1985; Ghodsian and Power, 1987; Bagnall, 1991). Ghodsian and Power reported on data analysed from a sample of sixteen year olds who were followed up again at twenty-three years of age. Their results showed that those teenagers who had reported heavier levels of consumption per week (more than 50 units for males; more than 35 units for females) were more likely also to be drinking heavily at twenty-three years. In contrast, Bagnall (1991) found no association between those individuals demonstrating frequent drinking at sixteen years and those who were drinking frequently at twenty-three years. A similar lack of association was reported by Plant, Peck and Samuel (1985). These authors examined a sample of fifteen to sixteen year olds and then sought them for re-interview four years later, when subjects were aged nineteen and twenty years. Just over 92 per cent of the original sample were re-interviewed. While they found that heavy drinking at fifteen to sixteen years was not predictive of heavy drinking at a later age, they did find that the young heavy drinkers were subsequently more likely than other teenagers to use illicit drugs. Finally, a comprehensive review by Fillmore (1988) also indicates that there is little continuity over time with regard to these early drinking patterns.

Adverse consequences of drinking

It should be noted that the majority of drink-related problems among adolescents are associated with the acute effects of intoxication as opposed to more chronic forms of abuse (Fisher *et al.*, 1987). As May (1992) points out, the exact relationship between levels of alcohol consumption and acute alcohol-related problems cannot always be easily defined. For example, the effects that a certain amount of alcohol will have upon an individual are likely to differ according to whether that person is male or female. Similarly, alcohol will have a differential effect on individuals of differing weight.

Acute negative consequences

Several studies have attempted to ascertain the frequency with which young drinkers experience negative consequences from their drinking. In Bagnall's study (1988) 19 per cent of subjects claimed to have experienced one hangover in the past six months, although a further 1 per cent claimed that this had happened more than four times within this same time period. A higher proportion of respondents (27 per cent) reported having had an upset stomach as a consequence of their drinking. Five per cent claimed that their drinking had caused them trouble with their parents or their school, and finally, 4 per cent had experienced an alcohol-related injury. Boys were also more likely than girls to report having experienced both positive and negative consequences of drinking, as might be predicted due to their overall higher rates of consumption. These negative aspects included being reprimanded by adults for drinking alcohol, feeling argumentative, feeling guilty about their own alcohol consumption and experiencing an alcohol-related accident or injury.

The incidence of negative consequences as a result of drinking was also examined by Plant, Peck and Samuel (1985). Of those subjects who had ever tasted alcohol, only 18.2 per cent had not experienced any of a series of negative consequences, ranging from intoxication to a variety of health-, social- and school-related problems. Furthermore, 20.2 per cent of males and 13.2 per cent of females had experienced at least one of six of the following serious consequences: having had four or more hangovers in the previous six months; having had a drink in the morning to steady nerves or get rid of a hangover; having been advised by a doctor to drink less; having had an alcohol-related accident or injury; having a shaky hand in the morning after drinking; and having missed a day at school due to drinking.

Drunkenness

Subjective reports of the incidence of drunkenness among teenagers are also widely documented. In her survey of thirteen to eighteen year olds in England, Hawker (1978) found that 68 per cent of the boys and 66 per cent of the girls reported having been intoxicated at some time during the previous year. Of these groups, 9 per cent and 7 per cent of boys and girls respectively had been 'very drunk' once within this time, while a further 16 per cent of boys and 10 per cent of girls reported having been 'very drunk' on more than one occasion during the year. More recently, Plant, Peck and Samuel (1985) found that of their Lothian region study group 70.4 per cent of boys and 61 per cent of girls reported having been drunk to a greater or lesser degree during the previous six months. Moreover, 36.4 per cent of all boys and 23.9 per cent of all girls in this sample said that they had been 'very drunk' within the past six months.

The common finding that the majority of adolescents have experienced intoxication to at least a mild extent is echoed in the findings of a national study by Marsh, Dobbs and White (1986). When this sample was subdivided by country (Scotland, England and Wales) and by age (from thirteen years to seventeen years), it was found that with the exception of the youngest group of Scottish girls, the majority of teenagers in each subsample had experienced some degree of intoxication. In the case of this particular group of girls, the proportion that reported having been drunk was 46 per cent.

More serious indices of drunkenness can be obtained from official records in which offences of drunkenness have been documented. The Home Office (1992) has reported that the numbers of known offences of drunkenness for England and Wales for the years 1989 and 1990 were 80,000 and 86,400 respectively. Four per cent of those found guilty of or cautioned for offences in 1990 were under the age of eighteen years, while a further 14 per cent were aged between eighteen and twenty-one years. The corresponding figures for the previous year were 5 per cent and 16 per cent. For both age groups, the majority of offences were for aggravated drunkenness. The peak ages for offending were nineteen to twenty years for males (around 1,010 per 100,000 population) and eighteen years for females (around 68 per 100,000 population). The rate of offending for those aged between ten and eighteen years was approximately 132 per 100,000 of the population. In comparison with figures over the past ten years, the percentage of male offenders under eighteen years has fluctuated slightly from between a maximum of 7 per cent of all known offences in 1985, to a minimum of 4 per cent in 1989 and 1990. With regard to figures for female offenders, these too have fluctuated only slightly, with a maximum of 9 per cent recorded in 1986, and a minimum of 5 per cent in 1981.

Accidental injury

Goddard and Ikin (1988) examined self-reports of driving under the influence of alcohol in a sample of 419 seventeen to twenty-four year olds in England and Wales. With regard to the male subjects in this age group ($n = 239$), they found that the majority (79 per cent) had not combined drinking and driving on any occasion during the previous year. However, 8 per cent had done so on three or more occasions, while a further 2 per cent reported that they regularly combined drinking with driving. Of the 180 females in the sample, 93 per cent claimed that they had not driven while under the influence of alcohol. Only 1 per cent reported that they had done so on three or more occasions, but again, a further 2 per cent reported that drinking and driving was a regular occurrence for them.

More objective data relating to the incidence of accidental injuries associated with the intake of alcohol have been reported by the British Medical Association (1986). Of the total number of recorded accidents for the previous year, sustained by sixteen- to nineteen-year-old-drivers, 30 per cent of these drivers had a blood alcohol count (BAC) in excess of 80mg/100ml – i.e. in excess of the legal limit for driving. The corresponding figure for drivers aged between twenty and twenty-four years was 42 per cent. The proportions for accidental injuries involving motorbike riders with similar BACs were 17 per cent and 26 per cent respectively. Although corresponding figures were higher among some of the older age groups, these statistics nevertheless are alarmingly high. However, a recent report from the Department of Transport provides more encouraging data concerning alcohol-related fatal road accidents (Department of Transport, 1990). The number of fatal road accidents occurring in the UK among drivers and motorbike riders with BACs in excess of 80mg/100ml, has declined dramatically over the last ten years or so. This is true of all age groups but is particularly marked among drivers under twenty years (Department of Transport, 1990). In a paper by May (1991), it is acknowledged that the issue of drinking and driving has received a higher and more weighty profile in recent years, both in terms of public awareness and law-enforcement strategies.

Comparisons with international data

When examining comparative data on international trends in youthful alcohol consumption, it is essential to acknowledge cultural distinctions in both national alcohol policies and normative drinking patterns. For instance, some South American and African nations condone (Mardigal and Miguez, 1985) or at least tolerate (Medina-Cardenas, 1985; Haworth, 1985) heavy drinking and even intoxication, and see these behaviours as integral to their culture. In contrast, the Scandinavian countries, particularly Iceland, are among the most conservative and least permissive with regard to adolescent drinking (Makela, 1984; Olafsdottir, 1985).

Early drinking experiences

The age at which adolescents in other countries commonly receive their first drink of alcohol is typically between thirteen and sixteen years (Ahlstrom-Laasko, 1975; Ahlstrom, 1987; Pandina, White and Milgram, 1991; van de Goor, 1991). In addition, in a comparison of data from twenty-eight countries, Ahlstrom (1988) found that boys commonly reported a slightly earlier age than did girls for the occasion of their first drink. Although the context in which these early experiences occur is usually the family home, this is by no means a universal phenomenon. For example, Irish and Northern Irish adolescents generally experience their first drink in the company of peers (O'Connor, 1985; Loretto, 1993), as do many Icelandic teenagers (Olafsdottir, 1985). In a survey of Swedish drinking habits, Hibbel (1985) also reported that while young people tend to drink wine in the company of their parents, spirit drinking often occurs outside the family setting, with friends.

Data concerning adult attitudes to permissible starting ages for drinking have been examined by Makela (1984). He found that adults in Iceland and Norway generally concurred in the belief that drinking with the family was permissible for eighteen year olds, whereas the median preferred age expressed by Finnish adults was lower, at seventeen years, and by Swedish adults lower still, at around sixteen years of age. Adults from all four countries felt that drinking with peers was permissible only at a later age, around eighteen and a half years, although again, those from Sweden reported a slightly lower median age (18.2 years). Less recent corresponding data from other countries indicate that French adults are considerably more permissive towards youthful drinking (Bastide, 1954; Freour *et al.*, 1969). In contrast, countries such as Mexico and Zambia (Roizen, 1981) reported adult attitudes that were considerably more conservative than those reported in the Scandinavian study.

Patterns of abstinence and consumption

The proportion of young abstainers appears to be higher for other countries in comparison with Britain. In the United States, Zucker and Harford (1983) reported that a little over 40 per cent of thirteen to eighteen year olds in an American national sample were abstainers. Scandinavian data also reveal higher abstention rates among young people than those apparent in the British survey data. A study of Swedish youth (Armyr, 1985) revealed that 31 per cent of males were abstainers, while 36 per cent of females were abstainers. This study also confirms the occurrence of higher abstention rates among females than among males, a trend that is consistent with the data from Britain and the USA (Zucker and Harford, 1983). Nor is the tendency for the proportion of youthful abstainers/non-drinkers to decline with age a uniquely British phenomenon (Schwartz *et al.*,

1986; Rashkonen and Ahlstrom, 1989). Moreover, among those young people who do drink, sex differences in the quantity and frequency of alcohol consumption in other countries also appear to be consistent with the British data. As a rule, boys drink more often and more heavily than girls (Rachal *et al.*, 1980; Zucker and Harford, 1983; Ahlstrom, 1988). As noted above, it is often difficult to conduct international comparisons of heavy drinking among young people as cultural perceptions of excessive drinking differ considerably. Nevertheless, the overall picture provided by US data (Pandina, White and Milgram, 1991) does indicate that these proportions (5–10 per cent) are somewhat similar to those reported in the British literature.

In conclusion, these data confirm that while acute alcohol-related problems are likely to be experienced by the majority of young people, more serious consequences appear to be restricted to a minority, despite the almost universal use of alcohol by this age group. Thus the recent emergence of 'moral panics' (Cohen, 1972; Dorn, 1983; May, 1992) concerning young people's misuse of alcohol, when set in the context of the scientific literature, is shown to be based upon the behaviour of a small minority of adolescents who do misuse alcohol, but whose activities have been highlighted and sensationalized by the media.

Social influences

Family

The issue of whether or not a young person will become a drinker, and if so, how much, how often, when and where this will occur, will be dependent upon numerous intrapersonal and external/ environmental factors. From a social learning perspective, these influences can be seen as the result of complex reciprocal interactions between the individual, the environment and the substance, i.e. alcohol (Akers, 1985). That is, in order to appreciate the extent to which one set of these factors will modify an individual's drinking behaviour, one must also acknowledge the influences of other sets of factors upon both the drinking behaviour itself and these initial factors. On a wider level, the way in which society as a whole communicates its culture to the individual is through the process of socialization. During infancy and early childhood, those social agents that are most salient for the child's immediate physical and emotional requirements are likewise responsible for the socially orientated motivation and the development of primary socialization of the child. Invariably it is the family, or more specifically the parents, who fulfil this role as social models. Thus it would be expected that parents might have considerable influence as models for drinking, at least within these initial years of a child's development. Indeed in an early review of research in this area, Maddox (1970) was led to conclude that awareness of parental drinking habits provided the strongest and most accurate basis for predicting the alcohol-related attitudes and behaviours of adolescents. While this is no longer considered to be the case – Maddox's review had in fact preceded most of the now firmly established research into youthful drinking habits – familial influence remains an important, but more complex, issue.

On a general level, it has been suggested that families influence their offsprings' drinking, at least indirectly, in that they are initially responsible for defining an individual's socio-economic status and ethnic and cultural background (Zucker, 1976). On the other hand, studies of more direct or active processes of family socialization and how these relate to the use of alcohol or other psychoactive drugs by offspring have highlighted various factors which may contribute to and shape this process. These factors can be seen as falling into two categories: social/observational learning or the imitation/modelling of parental attitudes and behaviour, perceived or actual; and family-process influences, i.e. family structure, family support and family control.

Social/observational learning

Direct modelling theory states that the acquisition of a particular behaviour is a result of direct observation of the behaviour of significant role models and the subsequent modelling of that behaviour. Kandel, Kessler and Margulies (1978) have suggested that this process is relevant to the initiation of adolescent alcohol use. Barnes (1977) also proposed that various patterns of adolescent alcohol use could be understood in terms of direct modelling from parents. In support of this, Barnes presented evidence indicating that parental drinking patterns ranging from total abstinence to heavy use were correspondingly reflected in the drinking patterns of their offspring. She went on to propose that alcohol-related attitudes and behaviours of parents were the best predictors of youthful drinking patterns.

There is much evidence to suggest that such a relationship does exist in relation to adolescent initiation to alcohol and adult use of alcohol (Johnson, Schontz and Locke, 1984). For example, children of families where one or both parents drink are themselves more likely to drink (Rachal *et al.*, 1975; Mookherjee, 1984). Nor does this appear particularly surprising when one considers that in many cases parents are actively involved in the process of initiating young people into the use of alcohol. In contrast, other studies have failed to identify a similar association between parental drinking and offspring use of alcohol (e.g. Newcomb, Huba and Bentler, 1983). White, Bates and Johnson (1991) have argued that the majority of these examples of direct modelling effects failed to take into account the social processes involved. Thus, subsequent research has expanded upon the direct modelling theory and has taken into account the role of cognitive mediation in the imitation process (Mischel, 1973). These theories affirm the importance of modelling effects, but stress that their impact is limited to the extent that they 'influence the cognitive mediation, assimilation, and perceptual processes in the child, which themselves motivate behaviour' (Newcomb, Huba and Bentler, 1983: 714).

In a study designed to compare the direct modelling approach with the cognitive mediational approach, Newcomb and his colleagues examined maternal influence on children's drug and alcohol use in a sample of 662 children and their mothers. Information concerning mothers' personality and mothers' use of drugs was collected by way of self-report questionnaires, as was information concerning sons' and daughters' own drug use and perceptions of adult use. The results showed no effects of direct modelling between mothers' use of drugs and children's use of drugs. However, the results did support a cognitive mediational association between mother and child, in that mothers' use of alcohol and drugs did have an effect on children to the extent that maternal behaviour appeared to influence children's perceptions of general adult use of these substances.

Various direct and indirect parental influences have also been examined by Wilks, Callan and Austin (1989), not independent of, but in conjunction with, peer and personal determinants of adolescent drinking. These authors found strong evidence of parental modelling effects on a sample of 106 adolescents. Especially in the case of young males, perceptions of parental drinking and fathers' actual drinking were the best predictors of alcohol use. Although not the strongest predictor of female use, fathers' drinking did appear to exert some influence on daughters' use of alcohol, whereas mothers' drinking had no discernible impact. Joyce O'Connor (1978), also found evidence of a differential effect between paternal and maternal influences on adolescent drinking. While parental drinking habits appeared to have little impact upon their children's behaviour, parental attitudes, and specifically paternal attitudes to alcohol, were noticeably influential.

Indeed, in relation to parental attitudes and normative standards set by parents regarding alcohol use, there is much evidence to indicate that these have some influence on drinking by offspring (Biddle, Bank and Marlin, 1980; Casswell, 1982; Wilks and Callan, 1984; Wilks, Callan and Austin, 1989). Positive parental attitudes to drinking have previously been found to predict initiation into substance use (Kandel, 1982; Newcomb *et al.*, 1987). Moreover, O'Connor (1978) also found that perceived parental attitudes were more influential on adolescent drinking than a variety of other parental factors.

More recent data relating to these influences have been reported by Foxcroft and Lowe from Hull University (1992). In their study of 430 teenagers, these authors collected data on, among other factors, parental attitudes to their offsprings' use of alcohol, and parents' own use of alcohol. The data referring to both parental attitudes towards their children's use of alcohol and parents' own behaviour in relation to alcohol were based solely upon the reports – i.e. the perceptions of the offspring. With regard to modelling behaviour, these authors found that the heavier adolescent drinkers in the sample were more likely to report that one or more members of their family drank regularly. Similarly, abstainers and infrequent drinkers correspondingly reported less regular drinking among their family members. In addition, data from adolescents' perceptions of their parents' attitudes revealed that heavy drinkers were more likely to report that their parents were either disapproving or ambivalent towards their own drinking behaviour, whereas 'sensible' drinkers were more likely to report that their parents had moderating attitudes towards their children's use.

The role of social learning from parents in the context of alcohol use is thus clearly significant. Moreover, it is apparent that there are a variety of paternal and maternal influences, some of which are more influential than others. However the nature of these influences and the extent to which they affect subsequent use of alcohol in offspring will also depend on upon the individual's perceptions of his/her family both in general terms and in relation to alcohol use.

Family process

With regard to studies of family process, the possible contribution to the alcohol socialization process of a number of salient factors has been investigated. These factors have often been subsumed under more general dimensions, the most frequently used of which are: family support – e.g. cohesion, conflict, affection, warmth, trust, concern; family control – e.g. rules, discipline, permissiveness, adaptability; and family structure – e.g. family/parental intactness, divorce, absence of father (Barnes, Farrell and Cairns, 1986; Foxcroft and Lowe, 1991). The latter authors conducted a meta-analysis of thirty published articles dealing with adolescent drinking behaviour in relation to these three family socialization dimensions. Their results revealed that all three factors demonstrated a negative linear association with adolescent drinking behaviour. In other words, adolescents from home environments which were either less supportive, less controlling or less intact (i.e. both parents were not present) were more likely to drink more. In addition, the authors also found additional evidence of a possible curvilinear relationship in relation to family control, suggesting that high levels of control might also lead to heavy drinking in offspring.

Data from other studies have confirmed this relationship between family-process dimensions and adolescent drinking. However, the relationship between these factors is not always found to be linear. For example, Barnes, Farrell and Cairns (1986) found that both high and low levels of family control were associated with heavy or excessive adolescent drinking. A similar curvilinear relationship with degree of family control was also reported by Glynn (1981). In addition, it has previously been shown that the offspring of both problem-drinking and abstinent parents are more likely to develop drinking problems than offspring of parents whose drinking habits fall somewhere between these two extremes (Kissin, 1974).

In a subsequent study, Foxcroft and Lowe (1992) went on to examine family-process factors in relation to the use of alcohol by teenagers. Levels of family support were assessed by the Relationships Dimension subscales of the Family Environment Scale (FES) (Moos and Moos, 1986). Likewise, family control was measured by the System Maintenance Dimension of the FES. Their results supported the findings of previous studies: subjects who perceived low levels of family support were more likely to be heavy drinkers, as opposed to the moderate or higher levels of family support reported by abstainers, infrequent drinkers and 'sensible' (moderate) drinkers in the sample. Similarly, the heavy drinkers were more likely to be those who reported low levels of family control, whereas all other drinkers were more likely to report high levels of family control.

It would appear, then, that in relation to family socialization to alcohol use the more extreme behaviours at either end of the family-process dimensions are more likely to result in less effective socialization to alcohol use, whereas moderate degrees of family support and family control are likely to produce effective socialization. However, it is essential to stress the reciprocal nature of the interaction effects of these factors when considering data from studies examining one or more of these factors. That is, while social learning and family process may influence adolescent drinking, adolescent drinking may likewise influence the nature and extent of social learning and family-process factors. Research is currently being conducted on the interactions between social learning and family process factors in relation to adolescent alcohol use (Foxcroft, personal communication).

It should be mentioned that less work has been carried out on the role of siblings, in isolation from the parents, within the family-process model. In the previous study by Foxcroft and Lowe (1992), older siblings were considered in conjunction with parents when applicable, but were not treated separately. Of the few studies that have dealt with this issue the evidence is conflicting. Some have indicated a significant relationship between siblings' use of alcohol (Needle *et al.*, 1986), while others have not (Clayton and Lacey, 1982; Coombs and Paulson, 1988). It may be that the role of siblings in the process of socialization to alcohol is closer in nature to that of peers.

Peers

The transition from childhood to adolescence is one that is characterized by an expanding network of allegiances to multiple social groups to which individuals refer as frames of reference for social behaviour. Most notable among these groups are peers. For girls, these groups are also likely to include boys who are slightly older than themselves, but the main point here is that at this stage adolescents are generally likely to be mixing more with friends rather than with their parents. However, that is not to say that these groups necessarily replace parents as social role models. For example, Rosenberg (1979) found that throughout adolescence parents were considered more highly than peers in terms of interpersonal significance. More generally,

Greenberg, Siegal and Leitch (1983) also found no evidence to suggest that age was a significant factor in perceptions of parent versus peer relationships. In addition, in the specific context of alcohol use, it has been found that the increasing importance of peers during adolescence does not develop to the exclusion of (Kandel and Lesser, 1972; Brook and Brook, 1988), nor necessarily in opposition to (Margulies, Kessler and Kandel, 1977), parental influence. Both parents and peers will tend to reinforce cultural or local norms. However, children who stay at home may face fewer conflicts of interests than those who distance themselves from the control of the family.

Unfortunately, the concept of 'peer pressure' in relation to substance use has come to be synonymous with the idea of the individual as an innocent who is subsequently tricked and led into 'undesirable' activities by 'undesirable' others. As Glassner and Loughlin (1987) point out, this particular concept of peer pressure (i.e. 'bad company'), is not called upon to explain the group activities of adults, nor does it appear to be used in descriptions of the taking up of 'socially approved' adolescent behaviours. So why should this be such a popular explanation for adolescent drinking?

The role of peers in the context of drinking is undoubtedly an important one in that they typically form the environment in which young people engage in what is, essentially, a social activity. It is commonly found that increases in age are accompanied by a growing tendency for adolescents to drink in peer settings (e.g. Plant, Peck and Samuel, 1985; Marsh, White and Dobbs, 1986; Plant and Foster, 1991). This tendency to drink outside the parental home is in turn associated with increases in the consumption levels reported by adolescents (Harford and Spiegler, 1983; Plant, Peck and Samuel, 1985; Plant and Plant, 1992). The finding that heavy drinking occurs more frequently among peer groups than in home settings when parents or other adults are present has been confirmed by a number of studies (Davies and Stacey, 1972; Aitken, 1978; Harford and Spiegler, 1983; Plant, Peck and Samuel, 1985; Harford and Grant, 1987). In Harford and Spiegler's study (1983) conducted in the United States, the majority of students (51 per cent) reported drinking in both home and peer settings, although more drinking occurred in the latter environment. It was found that adolescents who drank both at home and in peer settings drank more frequently than those who drank exclusively with peers, probably due to greater ease of access to alcohol. However, the amounts of alcohol consumed by both groups were similar. Also within this group of home + peer drinkers, an increase in the numbers of heavy drinkers was noted between the ages of twelve to thirteen and fourteen to fifteen years. This increase coincided with an increasing tendency to drink at parties, i.e. outside the home, and a corresponding decrease in home-based drinking occasions. Moreover, there was little difference in the proportions of heavy drinkers (defined here as those consuming five or more drinks per occasion) between the home + peer drinkers and those who drank exclusively with peers. On the basis of these findings, the authors concluded that peer settings appear to 'exert their own impact regardless of whether the student has had exposure to home drinking contexts or not . . .' (Harford and Spiegler, 1983: 187).

It is important to note that for the majority of older adolescents these increases in consumption levels tend to approximate normal adult levels, and then become stabilized (Plant, Peck and Samuel, 1985; Marsh, Dobbs and White, 1986; Goddard and Ikin, 1988; Health Education Authority, 1989, 1990; Plant and Foster, 1991). Thus, taken together with Harford and Spiegler's results, this suggests that peer influences alone do not necessarily lead to the adoption of more reckless or more 'unsafe' drinking habits. Indeed, it may be the case that peers themselves exert controlling influences on drinking behaviour, in that while young people may experience minor drinking-related problems such as intoxication, nausea, etc., they rarely incur much more serious trouble.

Alternatively, it has been suggested that peers influence adolescent drinking more in terms of providing models for behaviour than by the setting of normative standards for alcohol use (Biddle, Bank and Marlin, 1980; Rooney, 1982). For example, Biddle and his colleagues (1980: 236) found that while the drinkers and non-drinkers in their adolescent sample were more likely to have friends who were also drinkers and non-drinkers respectively, peer sentiment concerning normative alcohol use in the context of the group did not appear to influence adolescent drinking. On the basis of such findings, these authors concluded that 'adolescent drinking is likely to reflect peer example, not peer norms'. Similarly, in a study by Wilks, Callan and Austin (1989) the results also suggested that for male adolescent drinkers there was evidence of some modelling in relation to how frequently their male friends drank and how adolescents perceived themselves as drinkers. Perceptions of their friends' drinking habits were internalized as their own preferences and norms, whereas friends' perceived norms appeared to influence only one single aspect of their drinking behaviour, namely their current frequency of wine consumption.

A number of studies investigating more specific aspects of peer group influences have also been conducted. For example, Aitken and Jahoda (1985) used quantitative and qualitative measures to examine various patterns of drinking in natural settings among groups of young adults in Scotland. In relation to consumption, it was found that drinkers whose companions consumed large amounts tended to drink more themselves and to show higher drinking rates. Indeed, the best predictor of consumption among males was the average amount consumed by companions. Other studies have confirmed that this tendency to drink more heavily when in heavy-drinking groups is more pronounced among heavier-drinking males (Cahalan, Cisin and Crossley, 1969; Cahalan and Room, 1974; Orcutt, 1991). Aitken and Jahoda (1985) also found drink-purchasing procedures to be fairly useful predictors of consumption. Those groups, typically of males, who customarily engaged in round-buying procedures, also tended to consist of heavier drinkers. This is of little surprise when one considers that females generally drink less than males (Plant, 1990). Thus, in the case of females, 'time spent in the bar' was found to be a slightly better predictor of consumption than was consumption by companions.

Finally in this same study, overt pressures to consume or buy alcohol were also examined. It is noteworthy in itself that during these observations such behaviours were rarely noted. These incidents, when they did occur, appeared more often among groups of apparently under-age drinkers (i.e. those under the age of eighteen), although more subtle pressures were reported by all drinkers in subsequent qualitative interviews. In addition, those individuals in groups where overt pressure to drink was observed did tend to drink more alcohol. These latter findings suggest that more overt peer pressures to drink may be more relevant in situations where initiation into alcohol use is being negotiated (Aitken and Jahoda, 1985).

Among other group variables that have been examined, size of drinking group has often been found to be significantly related to consumption levels (Plant *et al.*, 1977; Harford, 1983), although the nature of this association remains unclear. Conflicting findings have also been observed in relation to the effects of sex composition of drinking groups on levels of consumption (Dight, 1976; Rosenbluth, Nathan and Lawson, 1978; Aitken and Jahoda, 1983). In addition, more recent data from a Dutch study by van de Goor (1990) also suggest that male and female adolescents differ with respect to the type of influences that effect their drinking. Female consumption rates appear to increase in mixed-sex groups and groups that engage in round-buying procedures. While male consumption rates appear to increase when drinking occurs in large, all-male groups, situational aspects of their drinking environment such as drinking in discos, in bars where loud music makes talking difficult, or in bars with higher variation in the size of clientele, appear to account for increases in consumption rates to a greater extent. Finally, results from a Canadian study (Graham, 1993) suggest that drinking behaviour in public bars may also be influenced by the design of the premises and the characteristics of the bar staff.

In general, it is clear that adolescents display similar drinking behaviours and attitudes to those of their peers. Abstainers commonly report higher numbers of abstinent friends than do drinkers, and vice versa (Wilks, 1987; van de Goor, 1990). However, the question of whether these influences are the result of the individual adapting to his or her drinking environment or whether the individual has self-selected the environment remains unanswered, although it appears that the relationship is reciprocal. Studies such as those carried out by Biddle, Bank and Marlin (1980) and Wilks, Callan and Austin (1989) are important in that they have considered the possible influence of peers in conjunction with parental and personal determinants, thus providing a more accurate and comprehensive account of the extent to which different competing factors may exert their influence. In addition, studies conducted in more natural settings (e.g. Aitken and Jahoda, 1985; van de Goor, 1990) are able to examine more specific and more subtle aspects of the social environment in which drinking occurs. Data from both of these types of studies suggest that a more useful approach for interpreting influences involved in the uptake and use of alcohol in the context of adolescent drinking would be to consider these behaviours as part of peer interactions, rather than as the result of peer pressures (Glassner and Loughlin, 1987).

Media

In any present-day discussion of the impact of external influences upon the process of learning to drink, the role of the mass media must also inevitably be considered. In Britain today it is estimated that around 98 per cent of all households possess at least one television. Moreover, households in which more than one television set is owned are likely to be those with children. Official estimates from the

Broadcasters Audience Research Board (BARB) indicate that average viewing hours are increasing for all age groups. Young children aged from four to fifteen years probably watch more than three hours of television per day. Nor are these viewing times necessarily restricted to within the watershed hour of nine o'clock in the evening. Comparable figures have also been obtained for the United States (Wallack *et al.*, 1990). Thus, television can be seen as a pervasive and potentially powerful medium for observational social learning and the transmission of socio-cultural norms.

An examination of the types of programme children prefer to watch suggests that programmes aimed specifically at children do not necessarily feature highly among their favourites. Soap operas are generally the most popular type of programme for children aged ten to fifteen years, and for those aged four to nine years. Girls tend to watch more soap operas than do boys, who tend to watch more sports programmes (International Broadcasting Authority (IBA), Broadcasters Audience Research Board (BARB), Audits of Great Britain (AGB)). Moreover, content analyses of television programmes (Greenberg *et al.*, 1979; DeFoe, Breed and Breed, 1983; Hansen, 1985; Wallack *et al.*, 1990) have revealed that alcohol is used consistently and extensively in a variety of programme types. Movies made explicitly for television and evening soap operas tend to include the highest proportion of occasions in which alcohol is used. Indeed, two extremely popular British soap operas – *Coronation Street* and *Eastenders* – both of which are broadcast during prime-time viewing hours and both of which also regularly enjoy some of the highest audience figures – are centred around a local bar. In addition, other types of programme, such as situation comedies, theatrical movies and dramas, also contain a high proportion of 'drinking acts'. With regard to the power of this medium to influence drinking behaviour specifically, it has been postulated that such portrayals have the potential to: (1) influence expectations regarding the use of alcohol; (2) influence attitudes concerning the acceptability or appropriateness of alcohol use; and (3) motivate people to model drinking behaviours (Greenberg *et al.*, 1979).

The drinking behaviour depicted on television is routinely shown to be an extremely commonplace and sociable activity, while at the same time often depicting drinking behaviours which might otherwise be considered inappropriate. Examples of these include apparent under-age drinking, drinking before driving, or drinking before and/or during working hours (Breed and DeFoe, 1981; DeFoe, Breed and Breed, 1983; Neuendorf, 1985; Hansen, 1985). Rarely is any mention given to the more negative consequences of consumption (Gerbner, Morgan and Signorielli, 1982; DeFoe, Breed and Breed, 1983; Signorielli, 1987). When drinking-related problems have been tackled, these tend to be centred around the short-term consequences which are themselves often treated in a light-hearted manner. The suggestion of more serious and longer term consequences are rarely considered, although there are currently exceptions to this. Indeed, several current British soap operas (e.g. *Eastenders* and *Brookside*) have been acclaimed for their realistic and sensitive treatment of the issue of alcohol dependence.

More recently, research has also focused upon the types of drinking models provided by television. Studies in the United States (bearing in mind that many US programmes are frequently imported to Britain and elsewhere) have suggested that regular programme characters are more likely than others to be shown drinking, and that these characters are themselves more likely to be the 'good guys' (Breed and DeFoe, 1978), upper class, attractive and glamorous (Wallack *et al.*, 1990). On the other hand, while many British-made soap operas are based around the activities of more ordinary, and possibly more credible characters, the potential for viewers to relate to these models may cause similar grounds for concern. Another source of role models in relation to alcohol and tobacco use can be seen in the televised sponsorship by these industries of sporting individuals, teams and events. The Sports Sponsorship Advisory Service previously documented over twenty different British football league teams in receipt of alcohol industry sponsorship for the years 1981–2, while a total of 102 alcohol brand names were associated with sports ranging from such diverse areas as greyhound racing, angling and badminton.

While the ubiquitous portrayal of alcohol in television programmes has been well established and the nature of such portrayals well examined, less is known about the subsequent effects in relation to viewers' attitudes and behaviours concerning alcohol use. It is generally considered likely that a causal relationship does exist (Flay and Sobell, 1983), although studies which have dealt with this issue have generated a series of conflicting findings. For example, Sobell *et al.* (1986) conducted a study of programme effects on consumption among a sample of male college students, within the artificial context of an experiment. Various versions of a videotaped prime-time television programme were shown to subjects, i.e. those in which alcohol scenes in the programme were either included or excluded. The type of advertisement that accompanied these presentations was also systematically varied to include advertisement for either beer, non-alcoholic drinks or food. In an apparently unrelated second task, subjects were then asked to perform a taste rating of a range of beers. The results suggested that those subjects who had observed either the drinking scenes within the programme or the advertisements for beer were not directly influenced by what they had seen, in that their subsequent consumption rates were no different from those recorded for the other groups.

In contrast, experimental studies with adolescents and children have suggested that exposure to even short segments of programmes with high alcohol content can produce dramatic effects (Rychtarik *et al.*, 1983; Futch, 1984; Kotch, Coulter and Lipsitz, 1986). For instance, in the study by Kotch, Coulter and Lipsitz, it was found that the boys in the sample were more likely to state that the good effects of alcohol outweighed the bad effects, following the presentation of a 'drinking' video showing only positive or neutral effects of drinking. Moreover, when questioned before the actual experiment, all boys had previously expressed the belief that alcohol causes more harm than good. No significant effects were found with regard to the female subjects.

Unfortunately, the ability to draw general conclusions about actual behaviour from data derived from artificial conditions is an issue justifiably contested. In the study by Rychtarik *et al.* (1983) children were asked to choose the most appropriate drink for adults from a range of alcoholic and non-alcoholic drinks, following an episode of the popular US television series *M*A*S*H*, in which alcohol scenes were either included or omitted. Those children who had witnessed the episode containing the drinking scenes were more likely than the other children to select an alcoholic drink when asked to state adult drinking preferences. Whereas it has been shown previously that many young children are aware that adult consumption of alcohol is a normative behaviour (Penrose, 1978; Greenberg, Zucker and Noll, 1985), it could be argued that these children were reacting to cues implicit in the design of the experiment in terms of their desire to make sense of the study (Goodman, 1990). In other words, they were simply responding to the cues in the film (or why else would they have been required to watch it?) and thus their responses did not necessarily extend to their wider beliefs about adult use of alcohol in general.

This raises the question of the possible ways in which attitudes and behaviour may be influenced, of which there are currently two theories. The first is based upon 'social learning theory' (Bandura, 1986), and assumes that television provides models for imitating behaviour in much the same way as the cognitive mediational model does in relation to parental influences. That is, the behaviour of significant role models is observed, considered and then subsequently acted upon. The second theory is known as the 'cultivation theory' (Gerbner *et al.*, 1986). Cultivation theory postulates that viewers learn a set of 'facts' from television programmes which often do not coincide with reality. This knowledge then 'cultivates' the individual's broader perception of the world, which in turn influences his/her own set of values and behaviour. To put this into the context of television portrayals of alcohol, the viewer who observes the pervasiveness of alcohol on television may consequently overestimate the number of people who drink and the normality of such behaviour. This may foster or reinforce in children beliefs about behaviours which are at variance with those supported by parents and other family members. Such dissonance may be particularly great in relation to children raised in a non-drinking environment.

The differences between these two theories are important in terms of scientific investigation of the effects of television. Social learning theory implies that a relationship exists between specific programmes and individual beliefs and behaviour, whereas cultivation theory attempts to examine the cumulative effects of exposure on a broader level. If the findings of, for instance, Kotch and his colleagues (1986) are found to be reliable, then this represents evidence in support of the latter theory.

Unequivocal evidence in support of a causal relationship between viewing of alcohol portrayals and increased use of the substance is lacking. Very little research has been carried out in relation to programmes *per se*. However, more information concerning these effects is available from studies on the effects of alcohol advertising. In 1987, the total alcohol advertising expenditure for press and TV in the United Kingdom was £119.91 million. This was equivalent to 9.7 per cent of total advertising expenditure on consumer goods for the same year (Statistical Review of Press and TV Advertising, Legion Publishing Services; Quarterly Digest of Advertising Expenditure, Media Expenditure Analysis Ltd). These figures represent a real increase over the past twenty years, both in terms of alcohol advertising expenditure and in terms of the proportion of expenditure on alcohol advertising in relation to expenditure on all consumer goods. On the other hand, a number of controls have been introduced by those bodies responsible for controlling advertising conduct, which have placed certain restrictions on the form in which this advertising can take. In brief, the aim of such restrictions has been to ensure 'socially responsible advertising' by preventing the promotion of images of drinking that are considered 'harmful'. In 1979, the following guidelines were laid down by the British Code of Advertising Practice of the Advertising Standards Authority:

RULES

Young people
3.1. Advertisements should not be directed at young people or in any way encourage them to start drinking. Anyone shown drinking must appear over 21. Children should not be depicted in advertisements except where it would be usual for them to appear (e.g. in family scenes or in background crowds) but they should never be shown drinking alcoholic beverages, nor should it be implied that they are.

Challenge
3.2 Advertisements should not be based on a dare, nor impute any failing to those who do not accept the challenge of a particular drink.
3.3 Advertisements should not emphasise the stimulant, sedative or tranquillising effects of any drink, or imply that it can improve physical performance. However, references to the refreshing attributes of a drink are permissible.

Strength
3.4 Advertisements should not give the general impression of being inducements to prefer a drink because of its higher alcohol content or intoxicating effect. Factual information for the guidance of drinkers about such alcoholic strength may, however, be included.

Social success
3.5 Advertisements may emphasise the pleasures of companionship and social communication associated with the consumption of alcoholic drinks, but it should never be implied that drinking is necessary to social or business success or distinction, nor that those who do not drink are less likely to be acceptable or successful than those who do. Advertisements should neither claim nor suggest that any drink can contribute towards sexual success, or make the drinker more attractive to the opposite sex.

Drinking and machinery
3.6 Advertisements should not associate drink with driving or dangerous machinery. Specific warnings of the dangers of drinking in these circumstances may, however, be used.

Excessive drinking
3.7 Advertisements should not encourage or appear to condone overindulgence. Repeated buying of large rounds should not be implied.

Despite these concessions on the part of the media control bodies, public health campaigners consider such restrictions still to be too vague and insufficient, with many arguing for nothing less than a statutory ban. The objection most commonly raised against alcohol advertising is that it increases total consumption of alcohol, which in turn results in an overall increase in alcohol-related problems. However, econometric studies on alcohol sales have failed to produce unequivocal data to support these claims (van Iwaarden, 1985). A review by Smart (1988) has indicated that neither advertising bans nor restrictions on expenditures on advertising have any significant or consistent impact on sales of alcohol. Similarly, Smart argues that in general studies have failed to demonstrate that advertising *per se* has an impact on alcohol consumption. Furthermore, when young people's day-to-day exposure to advertising has been examined in relation to their consumption, researchers have found the impact of advertising to be 'meagre' (Strickland, 1983), or very minor in comparison to other factors such as peer associations (Smart, 1988). Looking at this issue from another perspective, one study has examined the effects of the lifting of a ban on alcohol advertising in Saskatchewan, Canada, which had been imposed for a number of years. No subsequent increases in sales for alcoholic drinks was noted.

Although Atkin and his colleagues (Atkin, Neuendorf and McDermott, 1983; Atkin, Hocking and Block, 1984) found no strong association between exposure to advertising and adult alcohol consumption, they did find a significant relationship between exposure to alcohol advertising and teenage consumption of beer and liquor. While it has been argued by the drinks industry that 'they do not design their advertising to convince people to drink more. Rather . . . they are trying to increase their individual shares in the existing market' (Eisler, 1983: 45), they do also acknowledge that younger adults are often the target of much of alcohol advertising. For as they state, these individuals represent a group that is looking to establish drinking preferences, as opposed to older adults, who have probably already done so.

The suggestion that these commercials may have a greater effect on young people than on adults has been supported by other research (Jacobsen, Atkins and Hacker, 1983; Neuendorf, 1987). Aitken, Leathar and Scott (1988) conducted loosely structured interviews with groups of Scottish children aged ten, twelve, fourteen and sixteen years. They found that although few of the youngest children mentioned advertisements for alcoholic drinks among their favourite commercials, for the older children these commercials tended to be among those first mentioned. In addition, among these older groups, children demonstrated a high degree of awareness concerning the more complex imagery associated with advertisements for alcohol. These included references to social class, gender and sociability stereotypes.

In a subsequent study by several of the same authors (Aitken *et al.*, 1988), this degree of awareness and appreciation of alcohol commercials among young people was reinforced. Of the 433 ten to seventeen year olds interviewed, only 7 per cent were unable to name a brand of alcohol that had been advertised on television, with the most common of those mentioned being brands of beers and lagers. In addition, only 6 per cent failed to identify at least one photograph of a televised alcohol advertisement, while just over three-fifths were able to identify four or more. In accordance with studies that have shown a high sense of 'morality' towards alcohol use (Jahoda and Cramond, 1972; Spiegler, 1983), the younger children in the sample were more likely to advocate a ban on alcohol commercials. However, a high level of appreciation of the format of alcohol advertisements was also indicated by the majority of children irrespective of age.

Also in this same study, differences in perceptions of drinkers in comparison with non-drinkers were examined. Bearing in mind that all drinkers in the sample would be 'under-age', at least in terms of drinking on licensed premises or purchasing alcoholic drinks, it was found that the drinkers were significantly quicker than the non-drinking children at identifying the brand imagery in the commercials, and were also generally more appreciative of them. On this basis, Aitken *et al.* argued that while it is still not possible to state categorically that televised alcohol advertisements cause children to start drinking, it would appear that they do reinforce 'under-age' drinking.

It is generally accepted in the opposing case of alcohol education, that although people's attitudes may be affected by relevant information, this does not necessarily lead to a corresponding change in their behaviours. Indeed, in a comprehensive review of media-based strategies in relation to alcohol education Blane and Hewitt concluded that:

> The effect of public information and education programs on alteration of drinking patterns is indeterminate, although it is generally felt to be slight. Research evidence is almost totally

lacking; all that exists are bits and pieces of information that are no
more than suggestive.

(Blane, 1977: 537)

The problem with much of the research evidence apparently confirming a link between media influences and drinking behaviour,
positive or otherwise, is the issue of the causal relationship between
the two. Specifically, in the Aitken study, it was the older children
who tended to be those already drinking alcohol and who were more
aware and more appreciative of alcohol commercials. It has been
confirmed by epidemiological studies that many children around this
age have already begun to drink within the legally sanctioned context
of the family (see the previous section on youthful drinking patterns).
Moreover, there are numerous factors which influence youthful
drinking. Thus it is more difficult to assess the possible contribution
of alcohol advertisements in reinforcing this behaviour.

In spite of, or perhaps because of, the confusion surrounding this
debate, there are still many who would advocate a total ban on
alcohol advertising. This is a difficult issue, probably further complicated by the fact that anti-smoking campaigners have enjoyed greater
success in the fight against tobacco advertising. However, the ban on
tobacco advertising should not necessarily be seen as official confirmation of the undesirable effects of advertising on the incidence of
smoking, but rather as a culturally symbolic and political reaction to
the general issue of the harmful consequences of tobacco use. A more
compelling demonstration of this can be seen in the policy banning
the televised promotion of distilled liquor or spirits while at the same
time allowing other types of alcohol advertising to continue. It might
thus be suggested that a ban on alcohol advertising altogether might
also be justified, again not necessarily as an acknowledgement of
the harmful effects of advertising, but rather as a wider symbol
of society's values in relation to alcohol use. The longer-term ramifi-
cations of such action might prove to be more positive in that at least
the current ambivalence of our society towards alcohol use would
cease to be such a confounding factor.

THE CURRENT STATUS OF ALCOHOL EDUCATION

One formal response to widespread concern about youthful alcohol
misuse has been seen in recent attempts to integrate formalized
alcohol education into the school curriculum. These initiatives come
under the more general remit of the provision of health education for

young people, by schools, to 'facilitate voluntary adaption of behaviour which will improve or maintain health' (Green, 1979: 162). Moreover, the number of alcohol education materials now available has increased considerably during the past twenty years, as indicated by Plant (1993) in her recently compiled guide to 'Alcohol Education in Schools'. Most of these are targeted at adolescents and teenagers in secondary (high) schools, although a comparatively small number have also been designed for younger children, college students, teachers and parents. The motives for directing alcohol education primarily at young people are twofold: first, there is the assumption that young people constitute a more vulnerable group in relation to alcohol problems, due to their lack of experience; and second, there is the common belief or at least the hope that primary intervention strategies will help to provide adolescents with the necessary skills to cope in later life (Bagnall, 1991).

Underlying theories

In contrast to the explicit abstinence message conveyed by anti-smoking campaigns, the goals of alcohol education are less definitive and often differ with respect to each other. As Jessor (1982) notes, these may range from the promotion of total abstinence, to the delaying of onset of use, to equipping young people with the necessary skills which will lead to the 'responsible use' of alcohol, whatever this may be conceived to be. To further complicate the issue, both the use of alcohol and the form in which this occurs can be influenced by numerous factors. It has been suggested that certain factors or combinations of factors may be differentially associated with various stages of drug use. For example, curiosity, peer pressure, price and availability have been linked with both the onset of drug use and continued use of these substances. Alternatively, problematic substance use appears to be more commonly associated with a range of factors relating to adverse social and psychological circumstances (Plant and Plant, 1992). Even so, these classifications remain tentative and as such are not intended to provide a definitive portrayal of the processes behind problem substance use, the aetiology of which remains extremely complex:

> There is no single cause of drug misuse. It is not even possible to say with any confidence what the main factors are. Many explanations have been offered: ready availability of drugs, personality defects, poor home background, peer group pressure,

poor relationships, lack of self-esteem, youthful experimentation and rebellion, boredom and unemployment. All of these factors probably play some part. But there is no convincing evidence that any one – or any combination – of these factors is of greater significance that the rest.

(Home Office, 1985, para. 1.8)

Consequently, the conceptual framework upon which alcohol education initiatives are based has differed accordingly. For the purpose of evaluation, a number of researchers have attempted to place these programmes within some form of coherent classification.

Tobler (1986) conducted a meta-analysis of 143 adolescent drug prevention programmes, and highlighted five categories which distinguished between the functional content of these programmes: 'knowledge only' – in which facts about the consequences of drug misuse only are presented; 'affective only' – highlighting the psychological factors which place certain individuals at risk for drug misuse; 'knowledge plus affective' – i.e. programmes combining the above two strategies; 'peer programmes' – including the teaching of skills to resist peer pressure and enhancing personal competence, as well as peer-led programmes; and finally 'alternatives programmes' – consisting of other positive activities as alternatives to drug use and/or to enhance personal skills and competence. A meta-analysis of functional content carried out by Bangert-Drowns (1988) identified similar categories to those identified by Tobler.

An alternative attempt at classification has been described by Hansen (1992), which is based upon what he calls the 'building-block theoretical concepts'. Using this basis for distinction, Hansen identified six groups of programmes: information/values clarification; affective education; social influence; comprehensive; alternatives; and finally incomplete programmes. Others have attempted to classify programmes according to their theoretical basis. For example, Bruvold and Rundall (1985, 1988) identified four types of component common to programmes: rational components; social reinforcement components; social norm components; and developmental components.

A more parsimonious classification which encompasses the above categories is offered by Moskowitz (1989). Moskowitz proposed that in general, educational approaches are based upon one or more of the following three behavioural change models: the knowledge/attitudes model; the values/decision-making model; and the social competency model.

The knowledge/attitudes model focuses specifically upon behavioural use of alcohol. Stated simply, this approach is based upon the premise that an increase in knowledge about the consequences of inappropriate use of alcohol will engender in an individual more negative attitudes towards misuse and, as a result, the likelihood of engaging in problematic behavioural use of alcohol will be reduced. Historically, the philosophy underlying information approaches has shifted in emphasis from that of abstinence and the reliance on authoritarian statements, one-sided presentation of information and fear-appeals (Blane, 1977), to the advocation of 'responsible use' of alcohol through the dissemination of facts about alcohol and alcohol use.

Alternatively, proponents of interventions which employ the values/decision-making model argue that attitudes and behaviours cannot be changed simply by increased knowledge, but that affective or emotional factors, which may be responsible for the uptake of substance use and subsequent patterns of behaviour, must also be taken into account. As such these programmes are structured around psychological theories of individual behaviour. The central tenets of this model include the belief that individuals who misuse substances possess impaired value systems and/or insufficient ability to make the correct decisions regarding their use of alcohol. Thus the aim implicit in these strategies is to reduce the likelihood of alcohol misuse by promoting successful processes of self-examination of, for example, their value systems regarding substance use and/or their ability to engage in responsible decision-making.

The final model, that of social competency, has been developed more recently. This approach leans heavily on theories of social learning developed by Bandura (1977), for example, and considers the individual within the social context of alcohol use. It assumes that the development of alcohol problems can be understood in terms of inadequate social skills on the part of the drug user. Thus, the strategies employed for addressing this problem have involved the modelling of appropriate health-promoting behaviours, the acquisition by the individual of the necessary skills to resist the social influences that result in alcohol misuse, and more generally the teaching of positive intrapersonal and interpersonal life skills (Moskowitz, 1989).

Evaluating the success of alcohol education

It should be noted from the outset that evaluations of the efficacy of individual alcohol education interventions are conspicuously few in comparison to the large number of such interventions which exist currently. Moreover, of those that have been documented, few evaluations have been conducted on a sound methodological basis, and invariably only short-term outcomes have been considered (Goodstadt, 1985; Moskowitz, 1989; Bagnall, 1991; May, 1991). The seriousness of this failure to attempt any form of evaluation in the case of most education initiatives is further compounded by the fact that what little evidence is available consistently reveals such interventions to be quite ineffective. These shortcomings are described in greater detail in the following sections, in which interventions are discussed in relation to their theoretical underpinnings.

Knowledge/attitudes model

The provision of facts about alcohol consumption and alcohol-related problems as the basis for educational strategies has been the most enduring and currently remains the most widely adopted approach throughout Europe and the United States. One of the major premises underlying this model is that those individuals targeted are unaware of the possible negative consequences of alcohol use. Not only is empirical support for this notion lacking, but as Hansen (1988) has stated, the evidence available suggests that the reverse is true. A review of the current literature on children's early alcohol cognitions presented in the following chapter provides overwhelming evidence that even young children are aware to some extent of alcohol and its effects, and are particularly aware of the more negative consequences of use.

Nevertheless a number of studies have shown pre-test or baseline levels of knowledge to be significantly enhanced, at least in the short term, following such interventions (Globetti and Harrison, 1970; Grant, 1982; Goodstadt and Sheppard, 1983; Tobler, 1986; Bagnall, 1991). Moreover, in Tobler's meta-analysis (1986), in relation to other outcome variables such as changes in attitude, use of drug, social skills and general behaviour, knowledge increases accounted for the greater proportion of programme success in three out of five types of programme – 'knowledge only', 'knowledge plus affective' and 'peer programmes'.

Although superficially such results appear supportive of

information-only techniques, the utility of increased knowledge in terms of subsequent changes in behaviour remains doubtful. As Grant (1982: 8) states in his review of seventy-eight alcohol programmes:

> those who tested for increased knowledge were seldom disappointed, whilst those which tested for changes in attitudes, behavioural intentions or current behaviour displayed far more ambiguous results.

Bloom *et al.* (1956) and more recently McGuire (1974) have postulated that knowledge as a learning outcome for behavioural change can be classified by a number of stages, involving initial exposure to the educational message, attention to the message, comprehension of the message, initial and sustained agreement with the message content, and finally behavioural changes in response to the message. While studies confirming increases in knowledge suggest that attention to and comprehension of the message is often successfully achieved, there is little evidence to indicate that sustained agreement (i.e. attitude change) and/or corresponding behavioural change also become(s) established.

Indeed, with regard to subsequent changes in attitude and behaviour following the provision of alcohol facts, there is little evidence of a causal relationship (Degnan, 1972; Richardson *et al.*, 1972; Smith, 1973; Hanson, 1980; Kinder, Pape and Walfish, 1980; Goodstadt, 1981; Wallack, 1981; Goodstadt and Sheppard, 1983). Furthermore, when subsequent changes have been reported, these have commonly been observed to be at best minor and at worse counterproductive, in that they may have increased experimentation with the substance (Stuart, 1974; Cooke, Wehmer and Gruber, 1975; Kinder, Pape and Walfish, 1980; De Haes, 1987).

In response to such disheartening findings, some researchers have examined more closely the possibility of contaminating influences on the impact of didactic messages, such as the methods by which materials are presented, the perceived credibility of the communicator of the message, and the use of fear-arousal messages. In his review of seventy-eight alcohol education programmes, Grant (1982: 6) noted that 'the more passive the mode of communication, the less impact it tended to have on any variables other than knowledge'. Programmes which placed a greater reliance on interactive educational techniques such as discussions, audio-visual aids, field trips, etc. tended to yield more positive results in relation to possible behavioural change. Furthermore, in a study by Caleekal-John and

Pletsch (1984), an interdisciplinary approach, in which information about alcohol was disseminated in the context of an environmental physiology course, produced an increase in knowledge, positive increase in responsible attitudes towards alcohol use, and to a less significant extent, a reduction in the incidence of negative behavioural consequences among participating students.

With regard to communicator credibility and message content, Fritzen and Mazer (1975) found no difference in subjects' attitudes in relation to the non-alcoholic or alcoholic status of the communicator, but they did report less positive attitudes to alcohol following a high-fear message, when these were assessed at a one-week follow-up. However, no corresponding changes in drinking behaviour were observed for any of the conditions. More recently, Williams, Ward and Gray (1985) found that knowledge of alcohol was significantly enhanced when the communicator was perceived by the target group to be credible, and when the message was low in fear appeal. However, no subsequent changes in attitude were noted.

In a unique exercise, Smart and Fejer (1974) contrasted the impact of low- and high-fear messages on subjects' attitudes towards marijuana (cannabis) and an imaginary substance. While no attitudinal differences were reported for marijuana following either of the two conditions, the high-fear message concerning the imaginary substance produced more negative attitudes towards its use among subjects. While this latter study is interesting in that it demonstrates the relative ease with which attitudes to objects of which we are completely ignorant can be shaped, its usefulness is limited in the present context. What it does perhaps emphasize, though, is the fact that changing attitudes and behaviour in relation to objects with which individuals are already familiar is an altogether more difficult task.

In conclusion, there is little theoretical or empirical evidence to support the belief that passive communication of facts about alcohol can achieve the desired aims of alcohol education. And yet incredibly, as Rhodes and Jason (1988: 22) state:

> Despite the questionable etiology of this approach, as well as over a decade of research indicating that information alone does not deter or decrease substance abuse, drug education continues to be the most widely used approach to preventing substance use.

Values/decision-making model

The progression from didactic approaches to those involving more interactive learning techniques has been accompanied by a shift in emphasis from the psychoactive substance *per se*, to the individual as a substance user. As a result, psychological theories of individual behaviour have formed the basis for values/decision-making programmes. The focus of these strategies has been the enhancement of an individual's self perception, self-esteem, personal values and coping and decision-making skills, both on a general level and/or with specific regard to substance use.

In a comparative study of three education interventions, Goodstadt and Sheppard (1983) examined the outcome success of (1) a knowledge-only programme; (2) a decision-making programme; (3) a values clarification programme. As expected, the first approach significantly enhanced baseline knowledge at post-testing. While the decision-making programme did produce greater understanding of the major general decision-making concepts, as demonstrated by responses to hypothetical situations, no changes in relation to attitudes and/or actual drinking behaviour were observed. Similarly, the values clarification programme was also found to be ineffective in terms of both current and future expectations of alcohol use.

In another comparative study, Schlegel, Manske and Page (1984) compared the efficacy of a 'facts-only' approach with both a 'facts + values' approach and a 'facts + decision-making' approach. The 'facts-only' programme led to a reduction in consumption among students both at immediate post-testing and when followed up six months later. In contrast, neither of the combined interventions appeared to influence students' consumption, suggesting that such approaches undermined the impact of the provision of a facts-only component.

More positive findings have been reported by Schaps *et al.* (1982). In an evaluation of a multi-substance affective programme dealing with marijuana and tobacco as well as with alcohol, Schaps *et al.* measured outcome success in terms of a number of variables: knowledge of drugs; attitudes to drug use; perceptions of peers' attitudes to drugs; perceptions of the costs and benefits of drug use; and finally actual drug use. Their results indicated that at least for a subgroup of younger females (twelve to thirteen), effective changes were found in relation to knowledge, perceptions of peers' attitudes and actual use of both alcohol and marijuana (but not for tobacco). Increases in knowledge were also demonstrated by the older males and females (thirteen to fourteen), with the latter also displaying a heightened awareness of the negative consequences of alcohol use, but no changes in actual drinking behaviour were noted.

In contrast, Hansen *et al.* (1988) reported negative outcomes following a decision-making programme in relation to alcohol, tobacco and marijuana use. These negative effects were found to be persistent even after one- and two-year follow-ups.

In general, data from meta-analyses (Tobler, 1986; Hansen, 1992) have confirmed this pattern of findings. Tobler (1986) found that as a group, 'affective only' programmes had an extremely poor outcome success, particularly with regard to actual drug use following intervention. (However, as noted previously, Tobler's programme classification was not structured according to the underlying behavioural-change model but to the functional content, and as such programmes in her 'affective' category may have differed somewhat.) Similarly, Hansen (1992) has suggested that on the whole such programmes appear to have a rather neutral impact on subsequent substance use.

In conclusion, there is scant evidence to indicate that rational consideration of the positive and negative aspects of substance use has much predictive value in relation to subsequent use (Huba, Wingard and Bentler, 1980). In addition as Moskowitz (1989) points out, little evidence exists to suggest that initiatives based on the decision-making model achieve much success with adolescents in relation to drug education specifically, nor more generally with regard to other social and moral values (Governali and Sechrist, 1980; Urbain and Kendall, 1980; Leming, 1980–1).

Social competency model

A more promising alternative to alcohol education has recently emerged in relation to the social competency model. This approach sets alcohol use and related problems in the social context in which they occur and thus considers the social influences associated with drinking. Such interventions have had considerable success in the context of tobacco education, both in the short term (Gillies and Willcox, 1984) and possibly in the longer term (Vartiainen *et al.*, 1986). There is much research to support the belief that social influences are associated with alcohol use and misuse. Moreover, it has been postulated that adolescent use of tobacco and alcohol share common determinants (Millman and Botvin, 1983). However, the abstinence goal implicit to tobacco education is markedly different from the 'responsible use' goal of much of the alcohol education literature, and as such provides a differential criterion for success.

Nevertheless, results from studies incorporating a 'social skills' approach, either separately (Hansen *et al.*, 1988) or in conjunction with other approaches (Botvin *et al.*, 1984a; Botvin *et al.*, 1990; Bagnall, 1991) have yielded more promising indications. In each of these studies, subjects who were involved in a social influences programme reported modest but significant changes in actual drinking behaviour in comparison to the control subjects.

Bagnall's (1991) education package incorporated components of each of the three behavioural-change models. Those subjects who had not been involved in the exercise were significantly more likely than those who had taken part to report having consumed alcohol during the previous seven days. Moreover, subjects in the former group were also more likely to report higher maximum levels of consumption than those in the latter group. Similarly, Botvin *et al.* (1984b) found that subjects exposed to a cognitive-behavioural intervention were significantly more likely than those of the control group to report less frequent drinking occasions, a reduction in the amount of alcohol consumed per drinking occasion and fewer episodes of drunkenness. Furthermore, in a one-year follow-up study following implementation of a cognitive-behavioural programme, Botvin *et al.* (1990) also found that additional factors such as peer-led activities and supplementary or booster sessions enhanced the likelihood of reduced alcohol use. Similar findings were also found in relation to tobacco and marijuana use.

In general, data from meta-analyses confirm that '. . . the most efficacious program for reducing drug abuse onset is a program that features social influences resistance training as a major focus' (Hansen *et al.*, 1988: 150). However, such findings must be put into perspective. While it is widely acknowledged that social influence programmes or programmes which rely heavily on this behavioural-change model are generally more successful than other programmes (Hansen, 1992), it should be noted that these so-called 'success rates' are still relatively low, and are based on relatively short-term follow-up evaluations only. Moreover, the variety of components involved in these programmes makes it difficult to identify whether this degree of success is due to the accumulative combination of programme components, or whether it is due to one or more specific components.

This highlights the fact that very little is known about how the processes of social cognition and social behaviour relate to each other (Ford, 1982), and more specifically how they relate to each other in the specific context of drug-related behaviour (Huba, Wingard and Bentler, 1980; Botvin, 1982; Jessor, 1982; Moskowitz, 1983; Braucht and Braucht, 1984; Snow, Gilchrist and Schinke, 1985). For example, the current widely held concept of 'peer pressure' which forms the basis for many social influence programmes remains contentious and is rather simplistic. As May (1991) points out, it takes no account of the notion of peer pressure as a restraint on alcohol-related problems. In order to develop more effective educational techniques it is essential to understand just how these social influences operate.

CONCLUSIONS AND IMPLICATIONS

Alcohol education programmes generally conform to one or more of the three behavioural-change models outlined above. The evidence to date indicates that programmes based upon the 'knowledge-only' model produce at best very minor changes and at worst may increase experimental use of alcohol, while programmes based upon the values/decision-making model appear to have negligible impact on subsequent alcohol-related attitudes and behaviour. While programmes incorporating components based upon the social competency model may represent a more promising alternative strategy, the level of success of these programmes remains disappointingly low, even in the short term. In light of this evidence it seems incredible not only that existing alcohol education materials should be retained, but also that more recently produced materials continue to adopt similar formats.

One of the major problems faced by educationalists lies in the definition of the goals of alcohol education, and the subsequent evaluation of success in relation to these goals. For example, abstinence as an objective is specific and unambiguous, and one which in theory can be observed relatively easily in terms of assessing behaviour. Delaying onset of use is also relatively easy to assess, although the appropriateness of either objective in relation to young people, of whom the majority already report alcohol use to a greater or lesser extent, is rather doubtful.

However, strategies designed to encourage sensible drinking are both difficult to put into practice and difficult to evaluate in terms of outcome. Most adolescents who drink do so infrequently and the amounts consumed are generally small (Bagnall, 1991; May 1992; Plant and Plant, 1992). As a result it is difficult to assess the positive impact of interventions promoting responsible use of alcohol when the baseline use of alcohol is commonly seen to be low. In these cases the goals of education may be interpreted as reinforcing and maintaining responsible use. Alternatively, education may have no impact, in that individuals through their personal experiences have already established for themselves guidelines for drinking which coincide with the responsible message of the education initiative. For example, it may be that an individual who reports having been very drunk and having experienced acute negative effects as a consequence may have been put off reaching that stage of intoxication again as a result of that actual experience. Indeed, there is evidence that some people feel this is the only way to learn about alcohol (Loretto and May, 1993). Finally, it is noteworthy that the studies described in this review tend not to distinguish between the subsequent drinking patterns of heavy drinkers and those of light drinkers in response to the educational message. This would seem to be an important oversight.

These findings also raise the issue of the optimum age at which to focus alcohol education. The majority of school-based initiatives are aimed at secondary school children in their early to mid teen years. As the review of young people's consumption (Chapter 1) previously indicated, the majority of children at this age report having had some experience of alcohol. The study by Smart and Fejer (1974) involving attitudinal change in relation to an imaginary substance, suggests that in situations where little or no knowledge of the substance exists it may be easier to influence attitudes. While the current study sets out to demonstrate that awareness of alcohol is apparent in very young children, the implication here is that interventions targeted at an age when early cognitions are being formed might achieve greater levels of success. This issue is discussed in greater detail in Chapter 9.

The standard of alcohol education programmes in terms of the extent to which they achieve their objectives will inevitably be restricted by the extent of our knowledge concerning the complex aetiology of alcohol-related problems. Until full comprehension of the interactive influences between the substance, the individual user and the socio-cultural context in which use occurs (De Haes, 1987) is attained, this success will remain limited.

3 The study

The two principal aims of this study were, first, to assess the extent of young children's knowledge, attitudes and to a lesser extent, their behaviour, in relation to alcohol; and second, to compare the current perceptions of young children with those previously described in a classic study conducted more than twenty years earlier (Jahoda and Cramond, 1972).

With regard to these aims, it was proposed to examine the following aspects of children's alcohol cognitions:

1 ability to recognize alcoholic beverages by smell;
2 attitudes towards adult drinking behaviour;
3 perceptions of the social norms relating to drinking behaviour among men, women and children;
4 the age at which children conceptualize alcohol as a distinct entity;
5 familiarity with the physical manifestations of drunkenness;
6 understanding of adult motives for drinking alcohol;
7 extent of direct experience with alcohol;
8 future orientations towards alcohol.

In addition, children's perceptions of tobacco use were also examined as follows:

1 attitudes towards adult use of tobacco;
2 perceptions of the social norms relating to tobacco use among men, women and children.

In relation to these aims, an additional objective of the study was to identify priorities for future research and health education with respect to young children and alcohol.

BACKGROUND METHODOLOGY

The study areas

The study was conducted in state schools in two regions of Britain. The cities of Edinburgh in Scotland and Birmingham in England were selected as fieldwork locations on an opportunistic basis. The city of Edinburgh is situated in the Lothian region, and is the administrative, geographical and financial capital of Scotland. Its population is roughly 434,500, 1.1 per cent of which are made up of ethnic minority peoples. Unemployment is currently at the level of 8.3 per cent. The city of Birmingham is located in the West Midlands of England, with a population of around 992,800. It is primarily an industrial city, the manufacturing industry being the major employer. The rate of unemployment for the West Midlands stands at 11.7 per cent. Birmingham also has the second highest concentration of ethnic minorities after the south-east region of England, with approximately one in fifteen of the population belonging to an ethnic minority group (Central Statistical Office, 1992).

Sample recruitment, selection and demographics

The cooperation of the Department of Education in Edinburgh and Birmingham Health Education Unit was established by letters and personal visits, at which details of schools' involvement in the study were discussed. The respective directors then contacted those schools which had provisionally been selected at this stage, notifying the head teachers of their approval of each school's involvement in the project. Subsequent personal meetings between the researcher and the head teachers of these schools were then conducted, during which final cooperation was secured. In all, eight schools participated: four in Edinburgh, Scotland; four in Birmingham, England. These schools were selected on a non-random quota basis, according to both religious affiliation and the socio-economic status of the catchment population. Accordingly, two 'middle-class' and two 'working-class' schools were selected in each city; each pair consisting of one Catholic school and one non-denominational school. None of the eight schools originally selected refused to be involved.

The target study group consisted of thirty children from each school, with equal numbers of boys and girls from each of three age groups – five and a half to six and a half years, seven and a half to eight and a half years and nine and a half to ten and a half years. This gave a projected sample of 240 subjects. No attempt was made to control for racial groupings. There were two reasons for this. First, it would have been extremely difficult to find sufficient numbers of ethnic minority children in the Scottish schools. Second, in terms of methodology, the size of the study group was too small to cope with the introduction of this additional variable. Moreover, this was not intended to be a nationally representative study. Finally, as no parental details were collected, it was not possible to assess whether those from different ethnic backgrounds had been brought up to adopt the cultural values of their race of origin or whether they were fully integrated into British society. Nevertheless, the likelihood that ethnicity did influence performance in this study will be discussed where applicable, specifically in cases where differences in the results were observed between English and Scottish respondents.

Class lists were obtained from each of the eight cooperating head teachers. Only one class per age group was selected as these generally contained sufficient numbers of children to allow for refusals, while at the same time minimizing the number of excess children who might be disappointed at their lack of inclusion when sampling procedures were carried out. Letters were then sent directly to the parents/ guardians of these children, explaining the study and giving them the opportunity to withdraw their sons and/or daughters from participation. This technique of recruitment of subjects by 'contracting out' rather than 'contracting in' has been used elsewhere (Plant, Peck and Samuel, 1985; Bagnall, 1988; Plant *et al.*, 1990; Plant and Foster, 1991). It has been suggested that the latter technique usually results in a much poorer response rate, due to lack of motivation rather than a desire not to participate (Jessor and Jessor, 1978). Very few refusals from parents were encountered, although in two schools a number of home addresses were found to be out of date, thus preventing contact with these parents.

Random sampling was conducted on those children whose parents had been contacted and who had not subsequently been 'contracted out'. Accordingly, the total number of girls and boys per class list was divided by five (i.e. the number of children required of each class). Depending on the resulting figure, rounded up to the nearest whole number (n), every nth child was then selected. For example, if there were thirteen girls in one class, every third child on the list was selected, although this would necessitate going through the list twice. However, it was not always possible to use this random procedure, as for several of the classes, the number of male and female children falling within the correct age range who were available on the day of testing was small. In these cases, every nth child was then excluded

Table 3.1 Study-group design

City	Age	Middle-class area				Working-class area			
		Catholic	Non-den			Catholic	Non-den		
				Boys	Girls			Boys	Girls
Edinburgh	5½–6½	3	5	5	5	5	5	5	5
	7½–8½	5	5	5	5	5	5	5	5
	9½–10½	5	5	5	5	5	5	5	5
Birmingham	5½–6½	5	5	5	5	5	5	5	5
	7½–8½	5	5	5	5	5	5	5	5
	9½–10½	5	5	5	5	5	5	5	5

until the desired number of children remained. An insufficient number of boys in the youngest age group was found in one school. This procedure resulted in a final study group of 238 subjects, as shown in Table 3.1.

Study methods

Although the design of the tasks in this study often differed from that adopted by Jahoda and Cramond (which is described in full in the following section), the nature of the tasks and the order in which they occurred in each session followed the same procedure, with one exception. The final task of the second session was introduced only in the present study. Thus, the test battery was as follows:

Session 1	British Picture Vocabulary Scale
	Recognition of Smells
	Judgement of Photographs (1)
	Perceived Likes/Dislikes (1)
Session 2	Judgement of Photographs (2)
	Perceived Likes/Dislikes (2)
	Concept task
	Drunkenness films
	Adult motives for drinking

With the exception of the British Picture Vocabulary Scale, each test in the battery was administered in the guise of a game-like activity. This was done for several reasons, which have been have been elaborated elsewhere. The testing of each child was carried out over two half-hour sessions separated by roughly four weeks. As a result, a small number of children failed to complete all the tests due to absenteeism at the time of the second session. All testing was completed in the autumn term, 1991. The Scottish children were tested by the author. The English children were tested by Ms Erica Coles, an infant-school teacher based in Birmingham (but with no prior contact with the children in the target schools), who was trained by the author.

DESCRIPTION OF TASKS IN SESSION 1

British Picture Vocabulary Scale

(See following section.)

Recognition of Smells

Rationale

This task measured one aspect of children's familiarity with alcohol. Children are able to glean information about alcohol from a variety of sources, ranging from the home environment (parents, other family members) to the school environment (teachers, peers), to the wider remit of the media. This particular task provided an objective measure of children's personal contact with alcohol.

Materials

Nine small jars, identical in size and appearance and each painted to obscure their contents, were filled with one of the following odorous substances: peppermint essence, disinfectant (Dettol), vinegar, whisky (Bells), coffee (essence), bubble bath, beer (Grolsch), perfume and tomato ketchup. The latter item replaced paraffin, which had appeared in Jahoda and Cramond's original battery of smells. However, it was felt that paraffin was not a suitable substance for inclusion in a task which required children to identify odours from unmarked bottles. Bubble bath was also used instead of soap liquid, as it was felt that this was a more commonly used substance and would therefore be more readily identifiable.

Procedure

The task consisted of two trials. On the first trial, the child was presented with each jar in turn and simply asked, *Have you smelt this before?* Only if the child answered yes, was he/she then asked, *What do you think it is?* Irrespective of whether his/her subsequent response was correct, the child was then encouraged to say something about the substance, i.e. *Where have you smelt it before? Who uses it? Do you use it? Do you like it?* Responses were recorded, but no feedback was given. In order to minimize the confounding effects of generally poor human ability to identify odours, a second trial was carried out according to the procedures adopted by Noll *et al.* (1990). Nine colour photographs of the substances were placed in front of the child who was told that these were pictures of what was in the jars and so would help him/her guess what he/she was smelling. These photographs remained on view throughout the second trial. Those odours which had not been initially recognized or which had been incorrectly identified in the first trial were then presented to the child a second time. Again, irrespective of whether or not the substance was correctly identified, the child was encouraged to say something about the substance and responses were recorded. Correct responses and close approximations to the non-alcoholic items, e.g. soap instead of bubble bath, were all categorized as 'correct'. Similarly, children's responses to the alcoholic odours were deemed correct if they applied any alcoholic label to the odour.

Judgement of Photographs (1)

Rationale

The aim of this task was to obtain an indirect measure of children's attitudes towards adult drinking. The examination of young children's attitudes poses a number of methodological difficulties. The process of reflective thinking is not common to young children (Livesley and Bromley, 1973). The introduction of an unfamiliar attitude object such as alcohol will further complicate an already difficult task. Furthermore, any method that relies heavily on verbal ability runs the risk of confounding verbal ability with the variable to be measured (Shantz, 1983; Berndt and Heller, 1985; Yussen and Kane, 1985). Therefore a non-verbal and indirect measure in which inferences about the attitude can be drawn from performance on apparently objective tasks constitutes a more suitable method of inquiry. The assumption here is that performance on an objective task may be influenced by the attitude, and that a systematic bias in performance on such a task will reflect the influence of the attitude (Cook and Selltiz, 1964).

Materials

These consisted of four training photographs and forty-eight experimental photographs (eight of which were duplicates and acted as controls for consistency of the responses). New photographs were taken for the specific purpose of this task, but they did replicate those previously used by Jahoda and Cramond. For each session, the four training cards and twenty-four experimental photographs were used. In the first session, each photograph showed either a man or a woman engaged in one of three types of activities: an alcohol-related activity (drinking whisky, drinking wine, or drinking a pint (for the men) and a half pint (for the women) of beer); a tobacco-related activity (smoking a cigarette or smoking a pipe (the latter applied only to photographs of men)); a neutral activity (e.g. reading a book, drinking milk, speaking on the telephone). The item 'drinking wine' had not been present in Jahoda and Cramond's set of photographs, but was included in the present set to represent an alcoholic drink which might be more likely than beer or whisky to be associated with female drinkers. In the second session, those same men and women engaged in an alcohol- or tobacco-related activity were then shown in a neutral activity, and vice versa. There were three random orders of presentation of the photographs in accordance with Jahoda and Cramond's format, details of which are shown in Appendix 1. The same photographs showing the man/woman drinking wine were also used to depict drinking whisky. As a result, children were systematically assigned to either the 'wine' category or the 'whisky' category, but not to both. In order to minimize the common tendency of young children to focus on the physical characteristics of people (Livesley and Bromley, 1973) and encourage subjects to concentrate on the activity, the photographs were taken in black and white, and showed only the side view of the men and women.

Subjects' responses were recorded by means of a response box consisting of four compartments labelled respectively: 'Like very much', 'Like a little', 'Do not like a little', 'Do not like at all'. To help those children who might experience difficulty with these labels, additional labels were also attached to each compartment: a large 'L', a small 'L', a small 'D', a large 'D' respectively, and each was accompanied by an appropriately happy or sad face.

Procedure

The task was performed over two sessions. In the first session, prior to the actual experiment, time was taken to familiarize each child with the procedure. Once familiarity was established and the four training photographs had been used, the experimenter told the child: *I am going to show you some more photographs, and each time, I want you to put it into the box that says what you feel about it.* In Jahoda and Cramond's study the child was further prompted with the statement *some are nice and some are not so nice*, in order to counteract a possible 'Polyanna effect' of the children calling them all 'nice'. However, in the present study it was felt that such a statement might encourage the child to say what he/she believed to be the experimenter's 'desired' response. The tendency for children to try to structure their responses to coincide with the perceived desired response of the experimenter has been noted in a paper by Goodman (1990). For this reason the prompt was omitted from the current study. Finally, as a further method of focusing the child's attention on the activity as well as on the sex of the person, a verbal description of the photograph accompanied its presentation – e.g. *Here is a picture of a man reading a newspaper.*

The second session, carried out approximately four weeks later, followed the same procedure as the first.

Perceived Likes and Dislikes

Rationale

The purpose of this task was to examine children's understanding of the social norms associated with drinking. That is, to discover children's perceptions of the 'normal' drinking behaviour of three social groups – namely men, women and children. Again, the inappropriateness of direct verbal questioning necessitated an indirect approach to this question. For this reason, the method of inquiry adopted was based on eliciting children's perceptions of activities that men, women and children normally like or dislike. On the basis of these perceptions it is possible to construe basic images of social norms held by the children.

Materials

These consisted of two sets of lists of activities generated previously by Jahoda and Cramond, each consisting of four training items, followed by twenty-four experimental items/activities appropriate to child, female adult and male adult roles – e.g. going to school, sewing on buttons, mending a car. Jahoda and Cramond's lists included four alcohol-related items: drinking beer, drinking whisky, going to the pub, being drunk. In the present study a fifth alcohol-related item – drinking wine – was included as an example of a less stereotypically male drinking item. Two smoking items – smoking a cigarette and smoking a pipe – were also included. In order to ensure the standardized presentation of lists in terms of intonation and length of pause between items, the lists were pre-recorded on to audio tapes, as in the original study. Both the lists and the order of the items within each list were systematically varied (see Appendix 2). In each list, four of the items were repeated to provide a measure of consistency of responses.

The task was carried out over two sessions. During the first session the lists contained no mention of the alcohol-related items.

As with the 'Judgement of Photographs' task, children's responses were divided into the like/dislike format. In the original study, Jahoda and Cramond designed an apparatus consisting of a closed box with the four response windows (labelled *Like a lot*; *Like a little*; *Do not like a little*; *Do not like a lot*). Beneath each window was a button which when pressed, simultaneously lit up the appropriate label and sounded a buzzer. However, in the present task responses were registered by means of a computer. During the task, four windows appeared on the computer screen labelled 'Like very much' (with a large 'L'), 'Like a little' (with a small 'L'), 'Do not like a little' (with a small 'D') and 'Do not like at all (with a large 'D'), and each containing the number of the keyboard key appropriate to each option. On the keyboard itself, matching labels (i.e. large and small 'L's and 'D's) were attached to four corresponding keys. Each time the child pressed one of these keys, the four windows disappeared and the letter corresponding to the child's response appeared on the screen, and was then replaced again by the four windows. Finally, four dolls – one adult doll of each sex and one child doll of each sex – were used to further orientate the children at each stage of the task.

Procedure

Prior to the main task, time was taken to train the child in the use of the computer and to familiarize him/her with the procedure. This was then followed by the presentation of the four training items. At the start of the main testing, a child doll of the same sex as the subject was placed in front of the child next to the computer, and the child was then told: *Now you are going to hear lots of different things that people do. I want you to tell me what things you think he/she* (pointing to the doll) *likes to do and what he/she does not like to do; and you just press the button that says what you think.*

When this first run was completed, the child doll was replaced by one of the adult dolls, who was described as 'a lady' or 'a man', and the same list was played again. This procedure was then repeated for the third and final time with the second adult doll. If any child appeared to have difficulty understanding the concept of typical men and women, the adult dolls were then described as 'just like other men/women' or if they still had difficulty 'a man/lady just like your dad/mum'. The child doll was always the first one to be used, as it was felt that this would be the easier part of the test and so would allow the child more time to become comfortable with the task, before going on to the more difficult stages concerning adult preferences. The man–woman woman–man sequence was then systematically varied.

DESCRIPTION OF TASKS IN SESSION 2

Judgement of Photographs (2)

(As described above.)

Perceived Likes/Dislikes (2)

(As described above. However in this session the alcohol-related activities were now included in the lists presented.)

Concept task

Rationale

This task was designed to examine the age at which children acquire an understanding of the concept of alcohol. A number of studies have shown that children can acquire a basic awareness of a concept without necessarily understanding the meaning of the term (Jahoda, 1959). For this reason direct verbal questioning is unsuitable.

Materials

The task consisted of three sections – an initial training section, the experimental section dealing with the concept of alcohol, and a final section included to reduce the salience of the alcohol theme. Thus, the materials used in the first section of the task were: an apple, an orange, a banana, some grapes, a pear, a lemon (fruit), and meat paste, chocolate, cheese, an egg, biscuits, a bread roll (non-fruit); in the second section, bottles of beer, wine, whisky and sherry (alcohol) and bottles of milk, orange juice, Coca-Cola and lemonade (non-alcohol); and in the third section, a toy pig, horse, sheep and cow (farm animals) and a lion, tiger, elephant and hippopotamus (wild animals). As popular brands tend to differ between Scotland and England, some of the foodstuffs and bottles of drinks differed accordingly, so that children were not faced with items they did not recognize, but with which they would otherwise be familiar.

Procedure

At the start of the initial section, children were told that they were going to play a guessing game. Two items of food, one a fruit the other a non-fruit item, were placed on the table in front of the child who was then told: *Here are two things to eat. I want you to guess which one I am thinking about.* Obviously at this stage the child can only guess. If the child pointed to or mentioned the fruit he/she was told that it was correct. If he/she chose the non-fruit food he/she was told that it was wrong. The child was then shown further pairs of fruit and non-fruit foods, the former being the correct response each time. This continued until the child either made five consecutive correct choices, or spontaneously mentioned the conceptual link, or failed to understand the concept after approximately ten trials. In the original study the number of attempts allowed for each child was sixteen. However, initial testing in the present study indicated that children understandably became demoralized or upset or simply bored after being told they were wrong on this number of occasions, so the limit was reduced. This was the only aspect of the 'Concept' task which differed from the format employed by Jahoda and Cramond. At this stage, the experimenter then replaced all the food on the table and divided them into groups of fruit and non-fruit. If the subject had previously failed to understand the fruit theme, he/she was then asked: *What is it that makes all these things (i.e. the fruit) the same as each other but different from this other group of things (i.e. the non-*

fruit)? If the child still failed to give the correct response, the experimenter then explained the groupings to him/her. Questions were then asked about the various foods: *Where have you seen them? Who eats them? Which have you tasted? Who gave you a taste? Which do you like?* These questions were included in order not to arouse children's suspicion as to the main aim of the study, when similar questions would be asked during the alcohol section.

The main experimental section immediately followed the 'fruit' task. All eight bottles of alcoholic and non-alcoholic beverages were placed at random in front of the child, who was now told: *I want you to put these bottles into two groups like we did with the food, so that one group of bottles is different from the other group in some way. I want the same number of bottles in each group.* Irrespective of the groupings he/she then made, the child was asked to explain why he/she had grouped them in this way. If the child had failed to group the bottles according to the alcohol/non-alcohol division, the experimenter then regrouped them according to this criterion, and asked the child if he/she could explain this subsequent grouping. As in the preceding section of the task, questions were then asked about all the different kinds of drinks. As well as the questions previously noted above, subjects were also asked: *Where were you when you had a taste? What have you been told or heard about these types of drinks? Who told you these things? Do you think you will drink these when you are older?*

The third section involving the toy animals, was conducted in a similar manner to the previous alcohol section.

Drunkenness videos

Rationale

This task examined the stage at which young children are able to recognize the physical manifestations of drunkenness. It was also designed to elicit information about children's knowledge of and attitudes towards drunks and drunkenness.

Materials

In Jahoda and Cramond's study, three black-and-white loop films designed to portray bodily and mental states were devised, although insufficient resources prevented a sound track being added to these films. However, because of the high success rate shown by their sample even without sound cues, e.g. slurred speech, it was decided that the newly made films in the current study would remain without sound. These films were constructed in the same way as the originals produced by Jahoda and Cramond, except that they were now recorded on VHS video and, for two of the situations, a version incorporating a female character was also made.

The task was divided into three phases, for the same reasons as those relating to the 'Concept' task, i.e. to provide a training film, and an additional film to reduce the salience of the alcohol theme following the main experimental presentation. The video in the first phase involved a young boy going shopping with his mother for a present. The target emotion in this film was happiness, and the sequence of events was as follows:

A   A young boy with his mother choosing a toy in a toyshop.
B   Boy taking toy to counter where shop assistant wraps it up for him, boy smiling.
C   Boy smiling as parcel is handed to him and mother and child head for the door.
D   Mother and child walking from the shop, boy smiling (close-up shot).

The second phase concerned the drunkenness theme. Two videos were made, one in which the drunk character was a man, the other in which the intoxicated character was a woman.

A   Man/woman in a public bar drinking whisky/wine and then picking up a glass of beer/wine.
B   Man/woman draining glass and stumbling from bar.
C   Man/woman staggering towards door of bar.
D   Man/woman staggering along the road (close-up shot).

The third set of films also had both a male and female version. The target state in these films was exhaustion.

A   Man/woman in gymnasium weight lifting/on exercise bike.
B   Man/woman slowing down, then putting down weights/getting off exercise bike.
C   Man/woman entering changing room and collapsing on bench.
D   Man/woman wiping brow and looking exhausted (close-up shot).

The films were reconstructed so that they could be played back in reverse chronological order, cumulatively – i.e. section D would be shown first, followed by sections C and D, then sections BCD and finally sections ABCD.

Procedure

Each child was systematically assigned to either the female videos or the male videos. Before the first film was shown the child was told: *You are going to see some films of people doing different things. I want you to watch them and tell me what you think the person has been doing.* Following the first section (i.e. D) of the training film, the child was asked: *What is the boy doing? What do you think he was doing just before?* and responses were recorded. The child was then told that he/she would now see what was happening just before the initial piece of film, and the next section was shown, i.e. CD. If the child had been unable to give a satisfactory answer to the first two questions, these questions were repeated, followed by further questions: *What do you think of him? Do you think he is nice or not very nice?* Then parts BCD were shown and the following questions were added: *How do you think he feels? Is he happy or sad? When do people usually look like that?* The complete film, i.e. parts ABCD, was shown only if the child had still failed to understand the theme.

The drunkenness film was presented in the same manner, although several additional questions were now included: *Have you seen anybody like that? Where did you see them? Has anyone told you about people like that? What did they tell you? Who told you these things?* Finally, both the exhaustion film and the accompanying questions were presented according to the same procedure as the previous two films.

Drinking Vignettes

Rationale

The aim of this final task was to investigate the development of children's understanding of adult motives for drinking alcohol in various social contexts. This task did not appear in Jahoda and Cramond's test battery, but was designed by Gaines and colleagues in the United States (Gaines *et al.*, 1988). It was felt that this test examined an important aspect of children's alcohol-related knowledge, the inclusion of which would give a more complete overall picture of children's knowledge.

Materials

Three short stories or vignettes were selected from Gaines *et al.*, depicting three different roles of alcohol: (a) calming influence after shock (of being in a near-miss car accident); (b) facilitation of social interaction (when meeting strangers); (c) celebration of a positive event (winning a prize). Gaines *et al.* chose these alcohol 'roles' on which to base the vignettes on the basis of evidence from Brown *et al.* (1980) and Christiansen, Goldman and Inn (1982), showing that these types of roles for alcohol could be differentiated by most twelve year olds. A further vignette was also produced by the author, which was labelled (d) consolatory drinking (after bad news). All four vignettes are given below.

Social Anxiety

Mr/Mrs Brown has been invited over to a neighbour's house to meet some people he/she does not know. Before leaving his/her house to meet the strangers, Mr/Mrs Brown drinks three glasses of beer/wine/ whisky.

Celebration

While listening to the radio in his/her car, Mr/Mrs Green hears the man on the radio say that he/she, Mr/Mrs Green, has won a large amount of money as a prize in a competition. Mr/Mrs Green pulls over to a nearby pub (public bar) and drinks three glasses of beer/ wine/whisky.

Escape

On the way home from work, Mr/Mrs Smith's new car was hit and badly damaged by another car, but luckily he/she was not hurt. When Mr/Mrs Smith finally arrives home, he/she drinks three glasses of beer/wine/whisky.

Consolation

As Mr/Mrs Gray is about to go home from work, his/her boss comes into the office and tells Mr/Mrs Gray that there is no longer any work for him/her to do, so he/she must lose his/her job. When Mr/Mrs Gray arrives home, he/she drinks three glasses of beer/wine/whisky.

Two dolls – one an adult male doll, the other an adult female doll – were used during the presentation of the vignettes to represent the protagonist. This was to help children to focus on what was essentially an abstract/hypothetical story.

Procedure

Each child was systematically allocated one of the four vignettes. Both the sex of character and the type of drink consumed in the vignette also varied systematically between male and female, and beer, whisky and wine respectively. Before the vignette was read aloud, the experimenter placed either the male or female adult doll in front of the child, who was then told: *I am going to tell you a short story about Mr/Mrs Smith (pointing to the doll) and I am going to ask you some questions afterwards, so listen carefully.* The vignette was then read aloud by the experimenter, after which the following questions were asked of the child: *Why do you think the man/woman had three drinks of beer/wine/whisky? How did he/she feel before having the drinks? How did he/she feel after having the drinks?*

Allocation of subjects to tasks

Within the study, several of the tasks involved more than one manipulation of their basic format. Those aspects that were to be manipulated between subjects concerned the random orders of presentations of items, the sex of characters and the types of drinks in certain tasks, and also in the case of the 'Drinking' vignettes task, the type of vignette. With regard to the projected study group, there were 240 children, consisting of 48 groups of five children belonging to each basic cell (e.g. subjects numbered from 1 to 5 were boys aged five and a half to six and a half, from a middle-class area, attending a Roman Catholic school in Edinburgh, subjects numbered from 6 to 10 were boys aged seven and a half to eight and a half, from a middle-class area, attending a Roman Catholic school in Edinburgh, and so on). In order to ensure a balanced allocation of subjects to each version of the task, taking into account the necessity of ensuring that at least roughly equal numbers of subjects with their demographic manipulations could be found, this allocation took place before the subjects were themselves allocated a subject number. Thus the questionnaires were numbered and the version of each task preordained before the random allocation of the five children within each basic cell was carried out. This is what is meant when, in the following sections, reference is made to the 'random allocation' of subjects to the various versions of each task.

In the following chapters, the findings of these tasks are presented. Various statistical procedures were used to analyse these results, using both the Statistical Package for the Social Sciences (SPSS/PC)

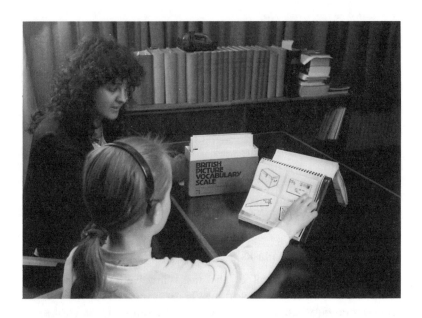

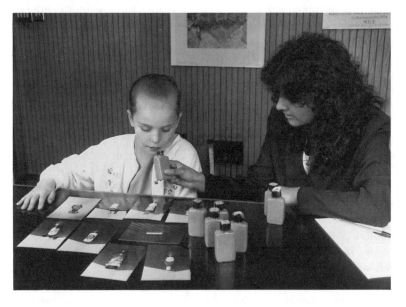

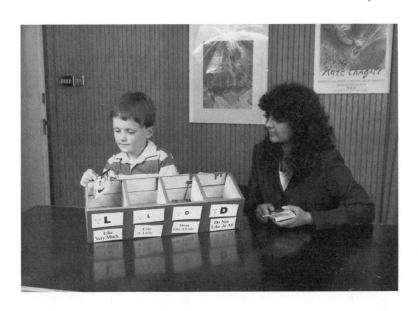

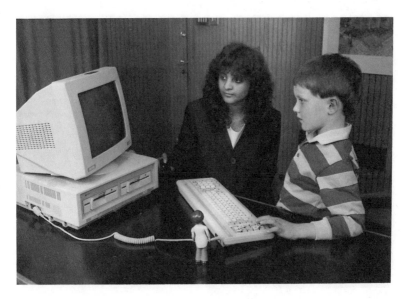

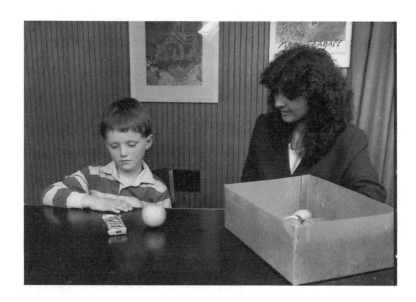

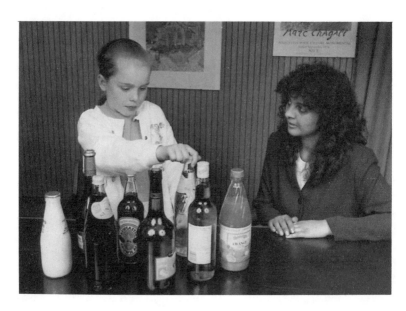

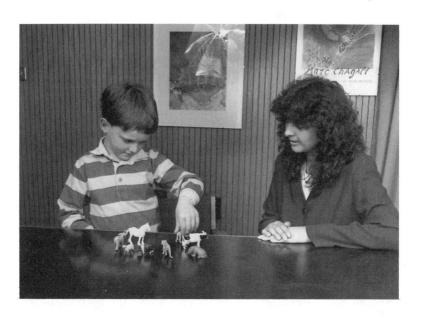

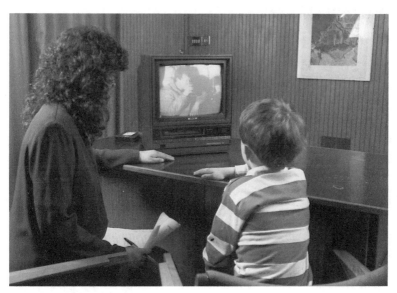

and GLIM (Payne, 1985). The following is a very brief outline of how these should be interpreted. The chi-square statistic, put simply, tests whether the observed frequency of respondents falling into a category is significantly greater or less than should be expected, based on the overall sample distribution. In the following text, if the probability (p) is less than 0.05 (e.g. $p < 0.001$), this indicates that the difference between what would be expected and what is actually found is significant. The same definition of statistical significance applies in the cases where analyses of variance are performed. Finally, both logistic regression and the loglinear regression analyses were used to estimate the effects of explanatory variables (e.g. age of subject, sex of subject, etc.) on dependent binary response variables (logistic) or multiple response variables (loglinear) – in other words, to predict the likelihood that a particular response will be given by certain categories of subject or as the result of certain type of influences within the task. For each analysis, a model is constructed which best fits the observed data, and the resulting log odds and 95 per cent confidence intervals for each variable in the model are given. The log odds can be exponentiated in order to produce the odds ratios for each variable.

THE MEASUREMENT OF SUBJECTS' VERBAL ABILITY

The English Picture Vocabulary Test (EPVT) was included in Jahoda and Cramond's study for two reasons. In the first instance, it would provide an enjoyable and relatively undemanding introduction to the main testing. Second, it would produce at least a rough measure of subjects' verbal ability with which to judge their performance on subsequent tasks. More recently, researchers in the United States (Greenberg, Zucker and Noll, 1985; Noll, Zucker and Greenberg, 1990) who have been conducting studies on young children's alcohol cognitions, have also employed the US version of this task – i.e. the Peabody Picture Vocabulary Scale to ascertain subjects' verbal proficiency. For these reasons it was decided to retain this task in the present study, although it was possible to use a more refined, up-to-date British version of this measure, entitled the British Picture Vocabulary Scale.

The British Picture Vocabulary Scale (BPVS) is designed to measure an individual's 'receptive (hearing) vocabulary for standard English'. It is stressed that the scale does not purport to be a measure of general intelligence, but that it does provide a measure of one major facet of intelligence, namely, vocabulary. Vocabulary has been found to be the best single indicator of school success (Dale and Reichert, 1957). However, in the present battery this test was included to provide a reference measure of subjects' cognitive development.

There were several additional advantages in using this particular test: minimal training of the examiner is required; scoring is objective; and standardized norms are available for the interpretation of the scores. Furthermore, the procedure is such that other skills such as reading and writing ability are not confounded with the specific skill to be measured. Finally, the test has no time limits, few verbal instructions and a cut-off point for errors, all of which ensure that subjects find it neither threatening nor demoralizing.

The Scale is a modified version of the Peabody Picture Vocabulary Test – Revised (Dunn and Dunn, 1981), which is itself a revision of the Peabody Picture Vocabulary Test devised by Dunn and Dunn in 1959. Although it has been used more commonly in the United States in areas of education, clinical and research testing, the BPVS has been modified to ensure its appropriate application in Britain. In addition, standardization has been carried out on a nationally representative British sample.

Numerous studies examining the reliability of the BPVS have been carried out, which have demonstrated conclusively that its reliability is stable for various specific subject groups. With particular reference to the short-form version of the test (the version used in the present study), corrected reliability coefficients ranged between 0.75 to 0.86 (median 0.80), for subjects up to the age of sixteen years. After this age, the higher ability of subjects is less reliably measured due to the small number of items in this test. However, the children in the present study fall well within this higher threshold.

With regard to the content validity, the stimulus words used in the test cover a fairly comprehensive range of word categories: actions; animals (parts and accessories); buildings (parts); clothing (accessories); descriptive words; foods; domestic fixtures; household utensils; parts of the human body; human workers and groups; mathematical terms; plants (parts); fruits and vegetables; school and office equipment; recreational equipment; transportation; and finally weather, geography and outdoor scenes. It should be noted, however, that the format of the test is such that words that cannot be depicted visually are necessarily excluded. In relation to construct validity, in both the Wechsler Intelligence Scale for Children – Revised, and the British Ability Scales strong correlations have been found between the vocabulary subtests in these tests and subjects' overall IQ scores (Wechsler, 1974; Elliot, 1982). Finally, a number of studies have revealed strong correlations between this particular measure and other measures of vocabulary and intelligence (for a review see Robertson and Eisenberg, 1981), providing confirmation of the criterion-related validity of this test.

Methods

Materials

The Scale appears in two forms: the short form (consisting of six training plates and thirty-two test item plates); and the long form (consisting of six training plates and 150 test item plates). The former was used in the present study. Each consecutively numbered plate or page consists of four numbered line drawings (i.e. the four drawings on each plate were consistently numbered 1 to 4). The experimenter is given a numbered list of words, with each word corresponding to one of the line drawings on each consecutive plate. As the test progresses, the words to be identified become more difficult or less familiar to subjects.

It should be noted that the short form of the BPVS is suitable for subjects ranging in age from two and a half years to eighteen years. Incorporated within the format of the test are standard age-based starting points which appear at various stages on the experimenter's word list. For this reason all subjects in the present study could be tested using the BPVS short form, although the starting point differed according to the age of each subject. Accordingly, older subjects commenced the test at a later, more appropriate stage in the word list, so that they would not get bored or over-confident by being asked to identify too many of the easier words at the outset.

Procedure

The training plates were presented initially, in order to familiarize the subject with the procedure. As each plate was presented, the subject's task was to identify the drawing, either by pointing to the drawing or calling out the appropriate number that corresponded to the word called out by the experimenter. As the main test progressed, these words became more difficult or less common. The test continued in this manner until the subject reached his/her ceiling item. This occurred when the fifth error within eight consecutive items was made. The subject's raw score was then computed by

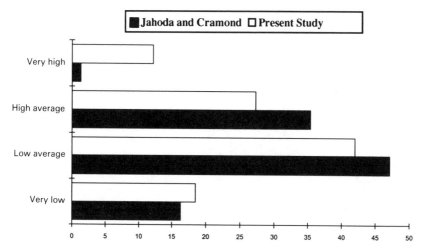

Figure 3.1 Between-study comparisons of BPVS scores

subtracting the total number of errors made from the number of the ceiling item. Conversion tables were then used to establish a standardized score for the subject. Percentile equivalents and vocabulary-age equivalents for the standardized score could also be calculated.

Results

Figure 3.1 shows the level of performance on the British Picture Vocabulary Scale for the whole sample, in comparison with the sample tested by Jahoda and Cramond. In the present exercise, the overall mean score for subjects fell into the 'low average' range at 96.83 (standard deviation = 17.28). The minimum score recorded was 61 and the maximum was 145, giving a range of 84.

Forward stepwise logistic regression was carried out in order to identify any differences which might have occurred between subjects. These results are shown in Table 3.2. The overall distribution of scores for this sample is very similar to that reported by Jahoda and Cramond for their sample, although in the present exercise a greater proportion of subjects recorded well above average scores. In both studies, middle-class children demonstrated superior verbal ability over the working-class subjects (in the present study increasingly so with age of child), thus validating a division between the two categories at least in this particular respect. The finding that subjects

Table 3.2 Subjects' performance on the BPVS (predicting the likelihood of a high score on the scale)

Parameter (reference categories in brackets)	Log odds	95% C.I. ↓	↑
Age (5–6 yrs)			
Age (2) 7–8 yrs	0.5114	−0.4316	1.4544
Age (3) 9–10 yrs	0.3995	−0.5367	1.3357
Ses. (m-c)			
Ses. (2) w-c	−0.7716	−1.7164	0.1732
City (Edinburgh)			
City (2) Birmingham	−0.7718	−1.3832	−0.1604
*Age *Ses.*			
Age (2) * Ses. (2)	−1.8710	−3.3786	−0.3634
Age (3) * Ses. (2)	−2.0140	−3.5816	−0.4464

from Birmingham performed less well than those from Edinburgh might be indicative of the higher proportion of ethnic minority subjects in the former group, a factor which should be borne in mind when interpreting the results of the following tasks. Although in the main experimental tasks the emphasis was on eliciting information by way of non-verbal techniques in order to minimize this risk of confounding verbal ability with the specific abilities to be measured, a number of additional direct questions did require a certain level of verbal ability.

4 Children's familiarity with alcohol and the concept of alcohol

THE RECOGNITION OF SMELLS TASK

Investigations of children's familiarity with alcohol have tended to concentrate on the assessment of children's visual identification of alcoholic beverages (Penrose, 1978; Jahoda, Davies and Tagg, 1980; Noll, 1983; Greenberg, Zucker and Noll, 1985; Gaines *et al.*, 1986; Miller, Smith and Goldman, 1990). Taken together, these studies have typically shown that even young children are able to recognize and identify various types of alcoholic beverage, either from photographs of bottles or from actual empty and unlabelled bottles. Furthermore, while some researchers have reported a significant relationship between parental drinking habits and various aspects of children's alcohol cognitions, including familiarity (Noll and Zucker, 1983; Greenberg, Zucker and Noll, 1985; Casswell *et al.*, 1985), others have found no evidence to suggest that such an association exists (Penrose, 1978; Jahoda, Davies and Tagg, 1980).

One possible explanation for these conflicting findings may be that there are two fundamental ways in which young children can become familiar with alcohol. One is by passive learning, which implicates external sources such as the media. Indeed, a study by Casswell *et al.* (1988) revealed that children cited television as the source of their alcohol knowledge more often that they mentioned their parents or siblings or any other source. The other is by active learning, i.e. direct experience which, at this young age, implicates sources in the immediate or home environment. It is apparent that visual identification of alcoholic beverages could be the result of either of these two processes. As a result of the confounding influence of information disseminated via external sources, few studies have been able to provide accurate, objective measures of the extent of alcohol learning that occurs specifically as a result of young children's direct experience with alcohol.

Incorporated into the design of Jahoda and Cramond's classic study was a task called the 'Recognition of Smells' task. This provided an objective measure of one particular aspect of knowledge that by definition resulted from children's direct experience of alcohol within their immediate environment. On the basis of their results, these authors were able to conclude the following: many children are familiar with alcohol from a very early age, and any age-related differences in performance could be attributed not to a lack of experience with alcohol but to an age-related ability to apply veridical verbal labels to odours in general.

Another study employing similar methods was conducted in the United States, with a younger group of children aged from thirty-one months to sixty-nine months (Noll, Zucker and Greenberg, 1990). However, to overcome the ancillary problem of verbal identification of odours encountered by Jahoda and Cramond's subjects, Noll and his colleagues introduced a second trial whereby children could identify the odours simply by pointing to a picture/photograph of the substance. With the younger children (thirty-one to sixty-nine months) in Noll *et al.*'s study group, identification was highly significantly related to age not only in the initial trial, but also following the assisted identification trial. Moreover, although performance on the non-alcoholic odours was significantly better than performance on the alcoholic odours in their sample, ability to identify non-alcoholic odours also displayed a similar age effect. It would appear that for children at this even younger age familiarity with a range of odours, especially alcoholic ones, has yet to become established due to limited opportunities for live exposure. Thus, when verbal identification was assisted in the second trial, persistent age-related increases in successful performance could now be accounted for by corresponding age-related differences in experience with alcohol. Despite the methodological differences between the two studies, the findings of both are strongly indicative of early alcohol learning taking place within the home environment.

The methodology adopted in the current exercise has been described in full in Chapter 3. However, in brief, this task consisted of two trials. In Trial 1 subjects were presented with nine odours in turn, and on each occasion they were asked simply whether they had smelt the odour before. Only if they claimed to recognize the odour were they then asked to try to identify it. Responses were recorded but no feedback was given to the subjects. In Trial 2, nine colour photographs of the substances were randomly placed in front of the subject. Those odours which had previously not been recognized or which had been incorrectly identified were now presented for a second time to subjects, who could refer to the photographs while attempting to identify these substances.

Results

The odours used in this task were of either alcoholic beverages or other substances. For the sake of brevity, these will be referred to as 'alcoholic' or 'non-alcoholic' odours respectively. Correct responses and close approximations to the non-alcoholic items, e.g. soap instead of bubble bath, were all categorized as 'correct'. Similarly, children's responses to the alcoholic odours were deemed correct if they applied any alcoholic-type label to the odour – i.e. the name of a different alcoholic beverage – or, for example, if they made more indirect references to alcohol such as mentioning that these were 'grown-up drinks'.

Identification of all odours

On this basis, a total of 1,013 (47.4 per cent) correct identifications were made on the initial trial. Only four children, from the two older age groups, successfully identified all the odours. Forty-nine children identified less than three of the nine odours (the arbitrary cut-off point established by Jahoda and Cramond, which categorized subjects as generally 'poor smellers', i.e. generally poor at verbal identification of odours). Chi-square comparisons between subjects who identified less than three odours and all other subjects revealed that the significant majority of subjects who fell into the former category belonged to the youngest age group, as expected ($X^2=30.6$; 2df; $p < 0.00001$).

Significant differences between the number of successful identifications for each odour were also found, as shown in Figure 4.1(a). Bubble bath was identified the most often and disinfectant (Dettol) the least often ($X^2=144.5$; 8df; $p < 0.00001$).

As expected, the inclusion of photographic cues in the second trial made a significant difference to performance for all odours. This resulted in an increase of over 30 per cent, to make a total of 1,671 (78.2 per cent) correct identifications. A total of sixty-one children (25.63 per cent) correctly identified all the odours presented, with the help of the cues. Chi-square analysis of subjects who identified

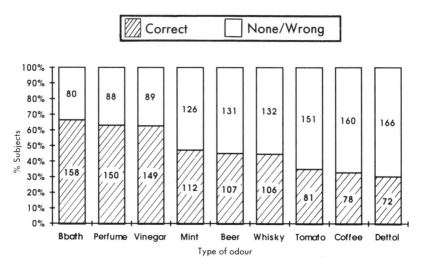

Figure 4.1(a) Identification of odours following Trial 1

all odours and all other subjects revealed that ability to identify all odours still increased significantly with age ($X^2=33.3$; 2df; $p < 0.00001$). Only ten children still failed to identify three or more odours, all but one of whom belonged to the youngest age group.

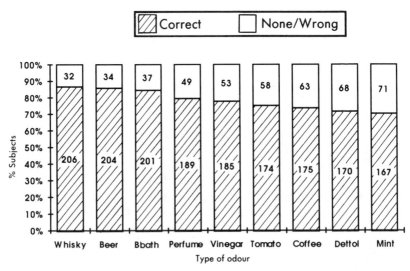

Figure 4.1(b) Identification of odours following Trial 2

Identification of the alcoholic beverage odours

Following the cued trial, the pattern of identification of the odours also changed. Whisky and beer became the odours most often identified, with mint now being identified the least often (X^2=43.33; 8df; p < 0.00001). Response rates for all odours on this second trial are shown in Figure 4.1(b).

With regard to the alcoholic odours, when these were analysed individually, there were no significant differences between the total number of correct responses for beer and the total number of correct responses for whisky, on either of the two trials. However, the number of children (n = 141) who labelled the odour beer 'beer' as opposed to any other alcoholic drink was significantly greater than the number of children (n = 54) who labelled whisky 'whisky' as opposed to any other drink (X^2=75.73; 1df; p < 0.00001), indicating that the term 'beer' was the subjects' preferred generic term for any alcoholic beverage. The separate response rates for each of the alcoholic odours are shown in Table 4.1.

Subjects' success in identifying the odours in relation to whether they had initially recognized them are also shown in Table 4.1. On the first trial, ninety (37.8 per cent) children initially claimed not to recognize beer and seventy-eight (32.8 per cent) claimed not to recognize whisky. However, on the second trial, seventy children from the first group and sixty-three children from the second group went on to identify correctly beer and whisky respectively. There were no significant differences in terms of ability to identify successfully these odours by name, between subjects who had initially claimed not to recognize the odours and those subjects who had initially claimed recognition.

Combining performance over the two trials, a total of 225 children (94.5 per cent) identified beer and/or whisky. One hundred and eighty-five (77.7 per cent) children identified both whisky and beer. Of this group, sixty-three (26.5 per cent) identified both odours without the aid of cues. Only thirteen subjects (5.46 per cent) failed to identify correctly either beer or whisky, five of whom identified less than three odours overall. These results are shown in Figure 4.2.

For each age group, identification of one or both of the alcoholic odours following the initial trial was as follows: five and a half to six and a half years = 38 (48.72 per cent), seven and a half to eight and a half = 54 (67.5 per cent), nine and a half to ten and a half = 58 (72.5 per cent). This relationship between performance and age was highly significant (X^2=10.62; 2df; p < 0.005). Following the second trial,

Table 4.1 Recognition and identification of beer and whisky

BEER

Recognition YES	Label given	Trial 1 −cues	Trial 2 +cues	Recognition NO	Label given	Trial 2 +cues	Total correct	None/wrong
(n=148)	Beer	70	19	(n=90)	Beer	52	141	
	Other	37	8		Other	18	63	
Total		107	27	Total		70	204	34

WHISKY

Recognition YES	Label given	Trial 1 −cues	Trial 2 +cues	Recognition NO	Label given	Trial 2 +cues	Total correct	None/wrong
(n=160)	Whisky	16	16	(n=78)	Whisky	22	54	
	Other	90	21		Other	41	152	
Total		106	37	Total		63	206	32

Responses falling into the 'other' category include occasions on which other types of alcoholic beverage were mentioned and those on which more indirect references to alcohol were made.

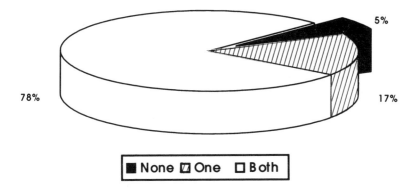

Figure 4.2 Identification of alcoholic odours

Table 4.2 Subjects' ability to identify alcohol following Trial 2 (predicting the likelihood of identifying beer and/or whisky by smell)

Parameter (reference categories in brackets)	Log odds	95% C.I. ↓	↑
Age (5–6 yrs)			
Age (2) 7–8 yrs	1.2080	−0.1660	2.5820
Age (3) 9–10 yrs	2.3330	0.2070	4.4590

these figures increased dramatically to 69 (86.25 per cent), 77 (96.25 per cent) and 79 (98.75 per cent) respectively. Forward stepwise logistic regression was conducted in order to ascertain whether age of subject and/or any other demographic variables were likely to have affected performance. The only significant between-subject difference to emerge was in terms of age. The youngest children were less likely than the oldest subjects to identify the alcoholic odours. These results are shown in Table 4.2.

Finally, the types of identification errors made by subjects were also examined, in particular the occasions where subjects identified non-alcoholic odours as alcoholic. Figure 4.3 shows the number of such misidentifications that were made for each odour. When these were crosstabulated with all other misidentifications for each non-alcoholic odour, i.e. when non-alcoholic odours were misidentified as

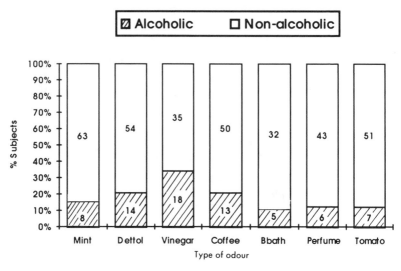

Figure 4.3 Label given to misidentified odours

other non-alcoholic odours, it was found that the odour vinegar was mistakenly identified as an alcoholic beverage on significantly more occasions than any other non-alcoholic odour ($X^2 = 15.12$; 6df; $p < 0.025$).

Discussion

The overall performance of the sample on the initial trial of the task was relatively poor. The percentage of successful identifications for all odours was only 47.4 per cent, with the older children significantly outperforming the younger children.

The human sense of smell has been referred to as 'the poor relation of the special senses' (Sumner, 1962). Although people are reasonably sensitive in detecting even weak odours and are able to recall past experiences when memory is triggered by a single relevant odour, human ability to accurately identify odours is extremely limited. The specific processes responsible for these limitations in human odour identification have yet to be pinpointed. Schab (1991) has suggested that these shortcomings may lie within one or more of three conceptualized processes involved in the course of such identification, namely the encoding of the odour, the activation of possible appropriate verbal labels in semantic memory, and the selection of the most appropriate label from those activated. In previous studies, tests of unassisted or 'free' identification of common odours have typically yielded low success rates of between 40 per cent and 50 per cent (Lawless and Engen, 1977; Cain, 1979; Engen, 1987). Thus the success rates of the current sample, following the initial 'free' identification trial (i.e. 47.4 per cent) fell within the expected range due to a commonly poor ability to identify odours. Furthermore, the age-related differences in performance on this initial trial could be attributed to developmental differences in verbal identification ability. For this reason further analysis of this set of results was not carried out.

However, it has been demonstrated that identification can be significantly enhanced when subjects receive some form of assistance concerning possible verbal labels. This assistance may take various forms: multiple-trial tests in which subjects are given feedback on their initial trial, self-generated labels (Cain, 1979); multiple-trial tests in which subjects are provided with veridical odour labels on the initial trial and then given corrective feedback (Cain, 1979); or finally, tests which incorporate a multiple-choice procedure (Cain, 1979; Engen, 1987). In order to ensure that the measurement of familiarity with odours was not being confounded with shortcomings in the general process of odour identification, especially with such young subjects, this study incorporated several tactics. As mentioned before, close approximations to the correct labels were also accepted as correct responses. However, in addition, a second trial was included using visual cues to aid the activation of verbal labels. As a result, the success rates following this second trial would provide a more accurate indication of the sample's familiarity with the odours. Moreover, any between-subject differences in performance could now be more justifiably interpreted in terms of corresponding differences in exposure to/familiarity with the odours.

When semantic memory was aided by visual cues on this second trial, the percentage of successful identifications increased dramatically to 78.2 per cent. Children were extremely successful at identifying alcohol. Indeed, whisky and beer were identified significantly more often than any of the non-alcoholic odours. When analysed separately, there was no significant difference between the overall identification rates for these two odours. However, the proportion of children who labelled beer as 'beer' was significantly greater than the proportion of children who labelled whisky as 'whisky'. This tendency to apply the label 'beer' to other types of alcoholic beverage has been noted in a previous study (Noll, Zucker and Greenberg, 1990) and suggests that for young children 'beer' is typically the preferred generic term for any alcoholic drink, rather than beer being more readily identified for what it is.

It has been demonstrated, as one would predict, that children are significantly more successful at identifying substances which are commonly encountered by children than they are at identifying substances used commonly or exclusively by adults (Noll, Zucker and Greenberg, 1990). The fact that in the present study alcohol – a substance used exclusively by adults – was identified significantly more often than odours more commonly encountered by children is difficult to explain. The reason for this may be that alcohol has a more distinctive odour compared to that of other substances. The finding that vinegar was mistakenly identified as an alcoholic beverage significantly more often than was any other non-alcoholic odour, would seem to support an explanation of this kind.

In relation to between-subject differences in familiarity, age of subject significantly affected performance on this task. The ability of the current sample to identify the alcoholic odours increased significantly with age in the initial trial, due to developmental differences in general verbal identification ability, as discussed above. However, when verbal identification was assisted in the second trial, almost 95 per cent of the sample identified at least one of the alcohol odours, 82 per cent of whom identified both. Although the majority of subjects who still failed to identify the alcoholic odours did belong to the youngest age group, it should be emphasized that only thirteen children, 5.46 per cent of the entire sample, fell into this category. On this basis it is possible to conclude tentatively that by the age of five and a half familiarity with alcohol is already sufficiently well established that, at least within this particular age range, further age-related increases in exposure to alcohol convey relatively little added advantage.

With regard to sex differences in performance, studies of general odour identification ability have found that females are typically more successful on such tasks (Koelega and Koster, 1974; Cain, 1982; Doty *et al.*, 1984). However, in the present study there were no significant differences in performance by sex for any of the odours, including the alcoholic ones. Neither Jahoda and Cramond, nor Noll, Zucker and Greenberg (1990) reported any gender-related differences in their studies. There were no significant differences in ability to identify either of the alcoholic odours by city, religion, nor in relation to socio-economic status or verbal intelligence of subjects, suggesting that early familiarity with alcohol is a pervasive phenomenon.

Data concerning parental drinking habits were not collected in this study, thus preventing comparisons to be drawn between parental use of alcohol and children's performance. Studies by Noll and Zucker (1983) and by Noll, Zucker and Greenberg (1990) have revealed a significant relationship between parental use and children's ability to identify alcohol by smell. Children whose parents reported heavier patterns of alcohol consumption (Noll, Zucker and Greenberg, 1990) and children of alcohol-dependent fathers (Noll and Zucker, 1983) were significantly more successful on the initial trial of the task, i.e. when no additional assistance was given, than children in environments where alcohol is present but less salient. However, following the second trial, there were no significant differences in performance. Thus, it can only be speculated that of the sixty-three children in the present study who identified both of the alcoholic odours without the aid of cues, some may have come from heavier drinking backgrounds.

Overall, the level of performance of the present sample was higher than that found in previous studies. In Jahoda and Cramond's study the success rates were as follows: six years – 39 per cent; eight years – 55 per cent; ten years – 61 per cent. Similarly, the success rates for the sample examined by Noll *et al.* (1990) were 69 per cent for those aged two and a half to four and 89 per cent for those aged five and a half to six years. With regard to Noll *et al.*'s study, this difference is likely to be due to the difference in ages between the two samples, as discussed above.

The rate of alcohol consumption in the UK has increased quite considerably in the intervening years since Jahoda and Cramond's study in 1972. While this might partly explain the greater familiarity with alcohol of the present sample, the differences in performance between the two studies are also probably largely due to differences in methodology. In the original study by Jahoda and Cramond, subjects received no form of verbal memory prompt during either of the trials. However, these authors did acknowledge that some children were generally poorer at identifying odours. To counteract this, they established a cut-off point whereby those children who had failed to identify three or more of the nine odours were excluded from subsequent analysis. Recalculating the success rates following this procedure, Jahoda and Cramond reported higher alcohol identification rates for each of the age groups: 74 per cent (six years), 69 per cent (eight years) and 71 per cent (ten years). As the youngest group also contained the highest number of 'poor smellers', the fact that this age group now showed the greater increase in performance should be considered more as an artefact of this procedure. Moreover, a second methodological difference between the two studies may also have been partly responsible for the differences in the results. If subjects in Jahoda and Cramond's sample claimed not to recognize the odour on the initial presentation, they were not given a further chance at identification. In the current study, a substantial proportion of children who claimed not to recognize the alcoholic odours on the initial trial successfully identified these odours on the second trial. Thus it is likely that even when the so-called 'poor smellers' were excluded from analysis, the success rates of Jahoda and Cramond's sample are probably an underestimation of the sample's true familiarity with alcohol.

To conclude, by about five or six years, many children are already familiar with alcoholic beverages to the extent that they are able to recognize and identify these kinds of beverages on the basis of smell alone. This awareness apparently begins to develop at an earlier age and increases with age up to about five or six years, at which time further age-related increases in exposure appear to lose their advantage. Previous research has tended to underestimate this familiarity, highlighting the difficulty in designing studies appropriate for young children. Often the methodological design of tests fails to take adequate account of the ways in which children perceive and react in these situations. As a result, it is often assumed that children are less knowledgeable with respect to alcohol than is the case. Furthermore, the early age at which this familiarity begins to develop strongly implicates the influential role of the family in children's early learning experiences in relation to alcohol. The implications of this will be discussed in the concluding chapter.

THE CONCEPT TASK

In the first part of this chapter it was demonstrated that young children are familiar with alcohol to the extent that they can identify various alcoholic drinks on the basis of smell. For very young children this familiarity may be as simple as knowing that such drinks are something that adults drink, whereas older children are more likely to be able to name specific alcoholic beverages. However, children's ability to recognize and name certain drinks does not necessarily imply that they have a conception of the possible social or behavioural implications of alcohol consumption (see Chapter 6). Nor does it necessarily follow that they understand the concept of alcohol as a distinct and logical class of drinks.

This latter point has been ably demonstrated in a study by Jahoda, Davies and Tagg (1980). Jahoda and his colleagues tested a group of 113 children aged between four and seven years. For the first part of the trial, subjects were simply required to name various pictures of unlabelled alcoholic and non-alcoholic drinks. However, on a second trial, these pictures were then divided into two – one group containing all the alcoholic beverages, the other containing all the non-alcoholic drinks – and children were then asked to explain the difference between these two groups. Jahoda *et al.* found that for the younger children (four and a half to six and a half years), ability to label pictures of alcoholic drinks correctly was not an indicator of ability to explain alcoholic/non-alcoholic groupings. Although roughly half of their younger sample could give the appropriate name to the bottles in the pictures they were shown, and roughly half were able to explain the subsequent groupings on the basis of an alcoholic–non-alcoholic division, the same children were not necessarily able to do both. On the other hand, with the older children in this sample (six and a half to seven and a half years), there was a significant relationship between those children who were able to name the bottles (i.e. roughly two-thirds of the group) and those who were able to explain the groupings.

In Jahoda and Cramond's original 'Concept' task, children were presented with a selection of bottles of alcoholic drinks (wine, sherry, whisky and beer) and non-alcoholic drinks (milk, lemonade, Coca-Cola and orange juice), placed at random on a table in front of them. The task required children to separate these eight bottles into two groups of four, so that one group contained four bottles that were similar to each other in some way, and the other group contained four bottles that were similar to each other but different to those in the first group. The children were then asked to explain the difference between the two groups. The correct response was to arrange the bottles according to the alcohol/non-alcohol division. If any child failed to group the bottles in this way, the experimenter regrouped the bottles accordingly and the child was given another opportunity to explain this subsequent reorganization.

Only 42 per cent of the youngest children performed the initial stage of the task successfully, with 40 per cent then giving a correct alcoholic-type explanation. However, following the experimenter's regrouping, a further 26 per cent were able to provide the correct explanation, giving a total of 66 per cent for this youngest age group. The older children were significantly more successful. Ninety per cent of the eight year olds and 96 per cent of the ten year olds successfully performed the alcohol grouping, with all but one child from each age group able to provide the correct explanation. Following the experimenter's regrouping, a further 6 per cent and 3 per cent respectively went on to complete the task successfully, giving respective totals of 95 per cent and 98 per cent for each of these two older age groups. The phrasing of children's explanations of bottle groupings also varied significantly with age. Not one of the youngest children mentioned the term 'alcohol'. In fact, only 11 per cent of the total sample had been able to do this, most of whom belonged to the oldest age group. The most popular way of expressing the groupings, for children of all ages, was to give the name of specific alcoholic drinks.

In brief, the methodology of this task in the current study was identical to that originally employed by Jahoda and Cramond. The task itself consisted of three parts: an initial training section, using fruits and non-fruits, to familiarize children with the demands of the proceeding task; the main experimental section, dealing with the concept of alcohol; and a final section using wild and domesticated toy animals, included in order to reduce the salience of the alcohol theme. For both the 'food' task and the 'bottles' task, care was taken to ensure that the item brands used were prototypical of their kind, i.e. those brands which would most commonly be associated with each particular product. In addition, as product brands tend to differ in popularity between Scotland and England, some of the foodstuffs and bottles of drinks differed accordingly, so that children would not be confronted with items which they might not recognize, but with which under other circumstances they would be familiar.

Results

The inclusion of the preliminary 'fruit' trial within this task was considered necessary in order to prime subjects for the more important, subsequent 'bottle-grouping' task. That is, it was important to ensure that children understood that physical characteristics such as shape, size or colour would be insufficient criteria for the groupings. The success rate of subjects on this initial trial was extremely high. Only eight children (3.5 per cent) failed to explain correctly the fruit/non-fruit distinction, even after all the items had been placed in the two appropriate groups by the experimenter and were displayed in this way in front of the child. However, as outlined in the methods section (Chapter 3), the principle behind the task was subsequently explained carefully to all subjects who had been unsuccessful, so it

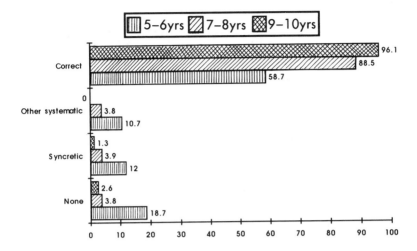

Figure 4.4 Subjects' groupings of the bottles

was not necessary to exclude these children from the main experimental section. Thus the performance, by age, of all subjects on the following 'bottle-grouping' trial is illustrated in Figure 4.4.

In total, 186 subjects (81.2 per cent) successfully dichotomized the eight bottles according to the alcohol/non-alcohol division, without requiring assistance from the experimenter. Eleven subjects (4.8 per cent) performed an alternative but nevertheless systematic grouping of the bottles and an additional thirty-two (14.0 per cent) failed to arrange the bottles at all or did so in a syncretic way. The majority of those children who failed to perform the correct divisions belonged to the youngest age group ($X^2 = 33.618$; 2df; $p < 0.00001$).

The majority of those subjects who had grouped the bottles correctly then went on to give an appropriate explanation based upon the alcohol concept. However, ten of these children subsequently gave an incorrect explanation. On the other hand, four subjects who had initially grouped the bottles in an apparently syncretic way then went on to give an alcohol-based explanation, *before* the experimenter regrouped the bottles. This would seem to indicate that while these four children were aware that the criterion for differentiating between the bottles was related to their alcoholic content, they may have been unfamiliar with one or more of the bottles with which they were presented.

For those remaining subjects who had failed to demonstrate satisfactorily an awareness of the alcohol/non-alcohol distinction, either

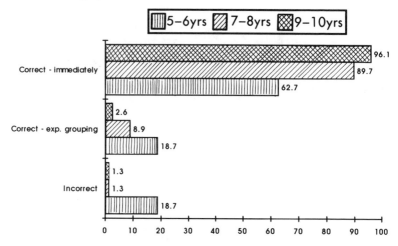

Figure 4.5 Subjects' explanations of groupings

in terms of their physical groupings and subsequent verbal explanations or solely in terms of their verbal explanations, the experimenter then placed the bottles into the appropriate groups. Each of these children was then given an opportunity to attempt to explain this new grouping. The results following this second trial, together with the amended success rates for the other subjects, are shown in Figure 4.5. Over 88 per cent of the total study group were now successful, with only 11.4 per cent failing to demonstrate an understanding of the alcohol concept.

Forward stepwise logistic regression was carried out in order to identify any between-subject differences in awareness of the alcohol concept. These results are shown in Table 4.3. Two significant findings emerged. As expected, the older subjects were more likely than the younger subjects to demonstrate an awareness of the concept of alcohol. In addition, children from Edinburgh were more likely than those from Birmingham to perform this task successfully. Furthermore, ability to perform the 'fruit' task was not a significant predictor of ability to perform this 'bottle-grouping' task.

Finally, having excluded the twenty-six subjects who had previously failed to demonstrate an understanding of the concept of alcohol, the way in which the remainder of the children phrased their explanations was examined. These results are shown in Figure 4.6. The most popular response overall was to mention the names of specific alcoholic drinks, with 46.3 per cent of the sample employing this technique. Only sixty-one children (30 per cent) mentioned the

Table 4.3 Ability to explain 'bottle groupings' (predicting likelihood of giving the correct explanation of the bottle groupings)

Parameter (reference categories in brackets)	Log odds	95% C.I. ↓	↑
Ses. (m-c)			
Ses. (2) w-c	0.01605	−1.2732	1.3053
Religion (Catholic)			
Religion (2) non-den.	−0.5377	−1.7651	0.6897
Age (5–6 yrs)			
Age (2) 7–8 yrs	1.8450	0.7186	2.9714
Age (3) 9–10 yrs	3.4980	1.3960	5.6000
City (Edinburgh)			
City (2) Birmingham	−1.7320	−2.8508	−0.6132
*Ses. * Religion*			
Ses. (2) * Religion (2)	2.1050	−0.0430	4.2530

term 'alcohol', while the remaining 23.6 per cent gave phrases containing more indirect references to alcohol – e.g. 'they're grown-ups' drinks'.

Of particular interest were those subjects who were familiar with the verbal concept of alcohol. For this reason, forward stepwise logistic regression was again carried out in order to identify those subjects most likely to be familiar with this term. As can be seen from Table 4.4, predictably, the older subjects were increasingly more likely than the youngest subjects to use the term 'alcohol'. In Edinburgh, those subjects with high scores on the British Picture Vocabulary Scale (BPVS) were more likely than low scorers to use the term 'alcohol'. However, in Birmingham, the effect of verbal ability on the likelihood of using this term was reversed. Finally, among Catholic subjects, those from working-class backgrounds were less likely than those from middle-class backgrounds to mention 'alcohol'. Moreover, this SES effect was increased among nondenominational subjects.

As the final 'animals' task was included only to reduce in subjects' minds the salience of the alcohol theme, the results of this section will not be presented here.

Discussion

The term 'concept' has been defined by Clark (1983: 789) as designating 'a set of properties that are associated with each other in memory and thus form a unit', and as such, 'the instantiation of a concept is a category'. Therefore, to categorize an object is to say that the object 'bears a particular relation to a particular set of ideas' (Neisser, 1987). Furthermore, categorization can occur at three different levels: superordinate; basic; and subordinate. This can be illustrated by taking, for example, the object 'dog'. The latter is a member of a basic level category, where animal is the superordinate category and labrador is a member of the subordinate category. Categories at the basic level are more readily recalled, more easily recognized and more easily named than categories at either of the other two levels. This is because the basic level is the one at which category members are most like each other and least like other neighbouring categories in terms of physical appearance, physical interactions and/or attributes. Studies have shown that children as young as one or two years already possess certain categories of objects (as well as situations and states) to which they can attach words as they acquire the necessary language (Clark, 1983). Moreover, it has been postulated that basic-level categories are the first kind to be acquired by young children. However, others have argued that for this to be the case it must be assumed that children's basic-level categories are the same as those of adults, which may not always necessarily be the case (Clark, 1978; Mervis and Mervis, 1982).

For very young children, the primary basis for categorization is the physical appearance of objects (Vygotsky, 1962). Evidence from

Table 4.4 Phrasing of explanations (predicting the likelihood of using the term 'alcohol' to explain the bottle grouping)

Parameter (reference categories in brackets)	Log odds	95% C.I. ↓	↑
Ses. (m-c)			
Ses. (2) w-c	−0.9665	−2.1843	0.2513
City (Edinburgh)			
City (2) Birmingham	1.7180	0.4802	2.9558
Religion (Catholic)			
Religion (2) non-den.	0.3639	−0.7291	1.4569
BPVS (low score)			
BPVS (2) high score	1.5380	0.1648	2.9112
Age (5–6 yrs)			
Age (2) 7–8 yrs	2.8760	0.7880	4.9640
Age (3) 9–10 yrs	5.0700	2.9460	7.1940
*Ses. * Religion*			
Ses. (2) * Religion (2)	−2.2600	−4.0872	−0.4328
*City * BPVS*			
City (2) * BPVS (2)	−2.3080	−4.0684	−0.5476

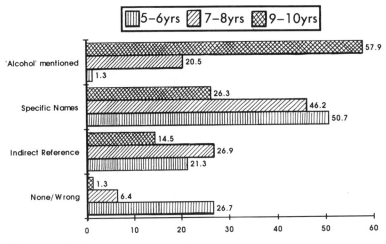

Figure 4.6 Subjects' phrasing of explanations

other studies that have examined children's ability to sort objects into conceptual groups has also indicated that young children may be more disposed to construct patterns or scenes with objects with which they are presented. However, while it may be the case that young children are more prone to categorizing objects in such ways, this should not be interpreted as implying an inability to perform alternative groupings (Keil, 1983). Markman, Cox and Machida (1981) tested this theory by asking children to sort objects into plastic bags, which would impede the construction of patterns or scenes, rather than on to separate pieces of paper which would facilitate this process. They found that under these conditions, children were less likely to construct patterns or scenes according to their personal preferences, and more likely to produce adult-like categories of objects.

In the current exercise, both the 'fruit' task and the 'bottle' task required subjects to organize subordinate-level members into their respective basic-level categories. While it has been mentioned that basic-level categories are generally more readily distinguishable, the present tasks were further complicated by the fact that the two sets of subordinate category members were not obviously similar to each other in terms of readily observable *physical* characteristics. Instead, for the tasks in the current exercise, subjects would have to be aware of the non-visible, internal attributes of the category members.

In addition to requiring subjects to look beyond physical characteristics in order to ascertain the shared properties of the objects, a further possible complication was the fact that neither the non-fruit items nor the non-alcoholic drinks constituted similarly distinct categories. For example, for the non-alcoholic drinks there was no other common property other than that they were all 'soft' drinks, i.e. they were not all fizzy drinks, they were not all 'healthy drinks', etc. Similarly, the non-fruit items shared no other immediately obvious characteristics apart from the simple fact that they were all examples of foodstuffs which were not fruit. In contrast, a task in which children were confronted with a mixture of dogs and cats for example, might be easier to perform successfully because it consisted of two more clearly distinct categories. However, the advantage of retaining this format in the current study was that it would be more difficult for children to perform the groupings successfully on the basis of the alcohol distinction, by default. The inclusion of the question asking children to explain their groupings could further ensure against the possibility of this happening unnoticed, if this were the case.

An examination of the performance of the current sample revealed that all but eight subjects were successful on the initial 'fruit' trial, either during the preliminary presentation of the pairs of fruit/non-fruit items, or once all these items were placed on the table in their two groups. For these eight children, time was taken to explain carefully the fruit/non-fruit distinction, and only when the experimenter was satisfied that the children had understood this did the main 'alcohol' trial then proceed.

As a result, over 81 per cent of the total sample went on to group the bottles accordingly, although it was a slightly lower proportion who subsequently indicated that their groupings had been selected intentionally on the basis of the alcohol distinction. In addition, subsequent to the experimenter's regrouping of the bottles, performed only where necessary, a further twenty-three subjects were able to explain the division correctly, giving an overall success rate of 88.6 per cent. As a point of interest, of those twenty-six children who failed to demonstrate an understanding of the concept of alcohol, four had been unsuccessful on the previous 'fruit' task. Nor was there any relationship between inability to perform the 'fruit' task and inability to perform the 'alcohol' task. As predicted, the youngest children were significantly less familiar with the concept of alcohol than were the older subjects. Nevertheless, over 81 per cent of this youngest group were successful. Similarly, children from Birmingham were less successful than their counterparts in Edinburgh. This may be due to the fact that the Birmingham sample contained a high proportion of children from ethnic minority back-grounds, within whose culture alcohol probably plays a more minor role. This difference between the two city groups also emerges in several of the other tasks, and will be discussed in the concluding chapter.

Examination of the type of explanatory phrases given revealed three categories of response. The first of these consisted of indirect references to alcohol, commonly containing references to the fact that these types of drinks were 'grown-ups' drinks'. The second category, and the one in which the greater number of responses fell overall, consisted of references to specific types of alcohol beverage, e.g. 'they're all beers'. The third and final response category con-sisted of all subjects, predominantly those from the oldest age group, who gave answers in which the term 'alcohol' was mentioned.

Age of subject again exerted a significant influence on responses to this question, with only one child from the youngest age group applying the label 'alcohol' to the grouping of bottles. In addition, children from middle-class areas were more likely than those from working-class backgrounds to be familiar with this verbal concept. Although verbal fluency did not emerge as a major single influence on responses, the fact that, as a whole, the working-class children in this study group demonstrated lower levels of verbal fluency than did those children from middle-class backgrounds may be indicative of some influence of cognitive ability. It may alternatively be the result of the way in which children of differing ages are informed about alcohol.

Developmental studies have suggested that adults typically use basic-level terms when describing objects to young children (Clark, 1983). For example they are more likely to use the word 'dog', rather than the superordinate term 'animal' or the subordinate term 'labra-dor', or 'apple' instead of 'fruit' or 'Granny Smith'. However, the fact that in the current study the majority of children mentioned the names of specific alcoholic drinks, i.e. subordinate-level category members, suggests that in relation to alcoholic drinks, adults may be more likely to refer to this essentially basic-level category by using the names of its more prototypical subordinate-level category mem-bers – e.g. 'they're all beers'. An alternative strategy that appears to have been adopted by a proportion of the children in this study is to apply a basic-level definition in terms of alcohol's function in relation to young children, e.g. 'grown-ups' drinks', and it is only as children become older that the term 'alcohol' then tends to be more com-monly applied.

Finally, in comparison with Jahoda and Cramond's findings, the younger children in the present exercise demonstrated a greater ability both in terms of performance on the bottle-grouping task and in terms of ability to explain the groupings. Moreover, a considerably greater proportion of subjects in the present study demonstrated familiarity with the label 'alcohol' as the defining term for the grouping. It would appear that children are currently learning more about alcohol at this young age than was the case twenty years ago, a trend which has been confirmed throughout this study, and one which might reasonably be assumed to be associated with the fact that per capita alcohol consumption has risen by 27 per cent in the intervening years (Brewers' Society, 1993).

5 Children's attitudes towards adult drinking and perceptions of related normative behaviours

THE JUDGEMENT OF PHOTOGRAPHS TASK

The majority of the tasks in this study were designed to examine subjects' knowledge on various issues relating to alcohol. However, another important but rather neglected facet of children's alcohol cognitions concerns their attitudes towards drinking behaviour. As part of their investigation, Jahoda and Cramond devised the 'Judgement of Photographs' task to obtain an indirect measure of subjects' attitudes towards adult drinkers. Their results revealed two particularly interesting trends. First, the youngest children in their sample displayed almost neutral attitudes towards drinkers, but as children grew older, attitudes became increasingly negative. Second, children of all ages tended to judge female drinkers more harshly than they did male drinkers. Using similar techniques on comparable samples from the United States and New Zealand respectively, both Spiegler (1983) and Casswell *et al.* (1985) have reported similar findings in support of this age-related trend. However, the tendency for children to be more condemnatory of female drinkers was apparent only in the Casswell study. That Spiegler found no corresponding trend within her sample is somewhat surprising in view of the fact that, in comparison with Britain, the United States contains a higher proportion of women who are non-drinkers.

Although information about the development of alcohol-related attitudes among young children remains limited, it would appear that there is a slower rate of development for alcohol-related attitudes than for alcohol-related knowledge. Moreover, the tendency for these early attitudes to be characteristically moralistic, becoming more so with increasing age of subject, appears to be a consistent trend. In contrast, studies of children above the age of ten years have shown that beyond this age, the orientation of attitudes towards alcohol reverses, becoming more positive during adolescence (Davies and Stacey, 1972; Aitken, 1978).

As has been discussed in Chapter 3, the study of young children's attitudes poses a number of methodological difficulties. Young children do not commonly engage in the process of reflecting upon their attitudes towards others (Livesley and Bromley, 1973). More generally, any method of testing children that relies heavily on verbal ability renders itself vulnerable to the risk of misinterpretation on two levels: the child's interpretation of the question and the experimenter's intended meaning; and the experimenter's interpretation of the response and the child's intended meaning. Therefore, a nonverbal and indirect measure in which inferences about the attitude can be drawn from performance on apparently objective tasks was adopted as the method of inquiry. This took the form of a series of photographs of men and women engaged in either an alcohol-related activity (drinking beer or whisky) or a non-alcohol-related activity (e.g. reading, eating, having a non-alcoholic drink), which were presented to subjects over the course of two separate testing sessions. In the second session, those men and women previously portrayed drinking alcohol or smoking were now engaged in a neutral activity, and vice versa. Children were required to place each photograph into one of four compartments of the response box – 'Like very much', 'Like a little', 'Do not like a little' and 'Do not like at all' – according to what they thought of it.

Results

In order to compare the results of the present study with those obtained by Jahoda and Cramond, scores were calculated according to the procedures adopted by the latter authors. A consistency check was also incorporated into this task in order to ascertain whether children's responses were conforming to a general pattern and were not just arbitrary. This was measured by means of four pairs of duplicate photographs. Consistency was thus defined as a pair of responses to the same photograph falling on the same side of the like/dislike division in at least three of the four possible matching pairs in each session. On this basis, the consistency of responses for each age group was as follows: six years = 66.66 per cent; eight years = 89.12 per cent; ten years = 90.66 per cent. These scores are slightly, but not significantly, lower than those reported by Jahoda and Cramond. As expected, the youngest subjects were more likely

Table 5.1 Subjects' attitudes towards adult drinking

	Age							
	5–6 yrs		*7–8 yrs*		*9–10 yrs*		*5–10 yrs*	
	Mean	*SD*	*Mean*	*SD*	*Mean*	*SD*	*Mean*	*SD*
Beer								
Men	42.60	11.91	49.81	12.41	54.17	9.99	48.87	12.39
Women	44.67	13.64	49.55	12.77	54.10	9.40	49.44	12.63
Both	43.63	10.82	49.68	10.95	54.00	8.35	49.11	10.93
Whisky								
Men	43.38	8.75	42.41	9.81	47.05	8.37	44.31	9.14
Women	45.09	10.76	47.94	10.73	55.77	9.53	49.69	11.22
Both	44.23	8.50	45.17	9.23	50.83	8.52	46.80	9.16
Wine								
Men	38.64	8.37	42.33	8.59	45.88	9.71	42.22	9.28
Women	43.86	10.04	47.66	11.26	52.82	11.38	48.02	11.40
Both	41.53	7.89	44.99	9.14	49.35	9.71	45.21	9.40

to be inconsistent in their responses, although not to the extent that their attitude scores then became invalidated.

Scores for the main part of the experiment were derived by assigning arbitrary values of 1 to 4 to the responses 'Do not like at all', 'Do not like a little', 'Like a little' and 'Like very much' respectively. Thus each photograph from both sessions had a score of between 1 and 4. Overall scores for each child were then generated by calculating the mean of the differences between the 'drinking' and 'non-drinking' versions of each photographed person. This provided each child with separate attitude scores for each category of drink and drinker, e.g. men and women drinking beer and men and women drinking *either* whisky *or* wine. The resulting pooled mean scores were then multiplied by 10 and increased by 40 simply in order to eliminate the decimal point and minus sign. This final computation produced scores ranging from 10 (indicating a very positive attitude towards drinking) to 70 (indicating a very negative attitude towards drinking), with a neutral score of 40. Table 5.1 shows the attitude scores of all subjects for all drinking items.

On the whole, attitudes towards adult drinkers were consistently negative, regardless of the type of alcoholic drink consumed and regardless of the sex of the person depicted drinking. However, beer

Table 5.2 Attitudes towards beer drinkers

	SS	DF	MS	F	SIG (P)
Between subjects					
Within cells	25880.83	146	177.27		
Constant	1046900.62	1	1046900.62	5905.82	0.000
Age (A)	8622.31	2	4311.16	24.32	0.000
Sex (B)	1815.10	1	1815.10	10.24	0.002
Ses. (C)	102.48	1	102.48	< 1	NS
City (D)	372.69	1	372.69	2.10	NS
Religion (E)	115.31	1	115.31	< 1	NS
BPVS (F)	160.22	1	160.22	< 1	NS
Within subjects					
Within cells	10370.83	146	71.03		
Sex of drinker (G)	21.87	1	21.87	< 1	NS
C * G	316.46	1	316.46	4.46	0.037

drinkers elicited more intense negative attitudes than did drinkers of the other beverages. In addition, subjects appeared to be more disapproving of female drinkers than of male drinkers.

In order to establish whether some subjects were significantly more likely than others to be negative towards drinkers, and to examine the possibility that the sex of the person drinking might also influence attitudes, separate multivariate analyses of variance were carried out for each of the three drinking categories. The results of these analyses are shown in Tables 5.2, 5.3 and 5.4. For the sake of brevity, only those interaction effects which were significant have been included.

Both age and sex of subject had significant effects on attitudes towards beer drinkers (see Table 5.2). Older children were more negative towards these drinkers than were younger subjects. Similarly girls were more judgemental than boys of beer drinkers. Gender of drinker exerted a significant effect on attitudes only when social class of subject was also taken into account, with working-class subjects being less disapproving than middle-class subjects of female beer drinkers compared to male drinkers.

When attitudes towards whisky drinkers were examined (see Table 5.3), the only main between-subject effect to occur was in relation to age of subject. Again, the older subjects demonstrated more negative attitudes than did the younger subjects. However, on this occasion, gender of drinker had a significant main effect upon subjects' attitudes. Female whisky drinkers were judged more harshly than male

Table 5.3 Attitudes towards whisky drinkers

	SS	DF	MS	F	SIG (P)
Between subjects					
Within cells	4416.82	41	107.73		
Constant	482286.61	1	482286.61	4476.92	0.0001
Age (A)	2367.30	2	1183.65	10.99	0.0001
Sex (B)	350.25	1	350.25	3.25	NS
Ses. (C)	0.11	1	0.11	< 1	NS
City (D)	174.83	1	174.83	1.62	NS
Religion (E)	336.37	1	336.37	3.12	NS
BPVS (F)	9.78	1	9.78	< 1	NS
Within subjects					
Within cells	1496.77	41	36.51		
Sex of drinker (G)	1720.02	1	1720.02	47.12	0.0001
A * G	493.90	2	246.95	6.76	0.003
F * G	153.38	1	153.38	4.20	0.047

whisky drinkers by subjects of all ages, although this was markedly so among the oldest children. When verbal fluency scores were taken into account it was found that higher scorers on this scale were also less disapproving of male whisky drinkers.

In relation to attitudes towards adults drinking wine (see Table 5.4), the older subjects were again more condemning of drinkers than were younger subjects. Children who scored highly on the British Picture Vocabulary Scale were also more disapproving than low scorers of all wine drinkers, but more so in the case of the women. Indeed, the female wine drinkers tended to elicit more extreme negative attitudes overall, in comparison to the male drinkers. Interestingly, the girls were even more disapproving than the boys of female wine drinkers. This is surprising in view of the fact that 'wine' was introduced into this task as an example of a less stereotypically 'male' drink.

Finally, two-sample t-tests were carried out in order to compare attitude scores obtained in the present study with those previously obtained by Jahoda and Cramond. Overall, the results of both studies were very similar. However, male drinkers were judged significantly less unfavourably by the eight-year-old (T = 2.61, p < 0.02) and the ten-year-old (T = 2.54, p < 0.02) children in the present study, compared to the children in the original study. Even so, the scores from the present study group remained quite clearly negative. There

Table 5.4 Attitudes towards wine drinkers

	SS	DF	MS	F	SIG (P)
Between subjects					
Within cells	6260.21	41	152.69		
Constant	438906.78	1	438906.78	2874.53	0.000
Age (A)	2611.23	2	1305.62	8.55	0.001
Sex (B)	346.20	1	346.20	2.27	NS
Ses. (C)	173.81	1	173.81	1.14	NS
City (D)	477.72	1	477.72	3.13	NS
Religion (E)	340.25	1	340.25	2.23	NS
BPVS (F)	791.84	1	791.84	5.19	0.028
Within subjects					
Within cells	1152.48	41	28.11		
Sex of drinker (G)	2273.31	1	2273.31	80.87	0.000
B * G	129.22	1	129.22	4.60	0.038
F * G	342.73	1	342.73	12.19	0.001

Table 5.5 Between-study comparison of attitude scores

	Age					
	5–6 yrs		*7–8 yrs*		*9–10 yrs*	
	Mean	*SD*	*Mean*	*SD*	*Mean*	*SD*
Present study						
Attitudes to men	41.65	8.24	45.35*	9.17	49.56[†]	8.45
Attitudes to women	44.55	10.05	48.40	10.40	54.25	8.98
Jahoda and Cramond						
Attitudes to men	40.84	8.50	47.49*	8.59	51.69[†]	9.65
Attitudes to women	44.09	7.82	48.61	8.37	54.40	9.25

* $t = 2.6067$; $p < 0.02$
[†] $t = 2.5851$; $p < 0.02$

were no significant differences between the two samples with regard to female drinkers. These results are illustrated in Table 5.5.

Discussion

The findings reported here are similar to those found by Jahoda and Cramond over twenty years earlier. As age of children increased so the negativity of their attitudes towards alcohol rose. However, male drinkers were judged slightly less unfavourably by the older children in the present study than by the older children in Jahoda and Cramond's sample. It had been predicted that the inclusion of the item 'drinking wine' might elicit less negative attitudes towards female drinkers. However, both female wine drinkers and female whisky drinkers were judged more harshly than their male equivalents, by all children. Even more surprising was the finding that female subjects were more condemnatory than male subjects of these female wine drinkers.

Attitude development

There are various ways in which attitudes can be formed: upon direct questioning; directly by means of personal experience and reinforcement; indirectly by classical conditioning, i.e. learning through association; or indirectly by social learning and observation. Social learning theory (Bandura, 1977) highlights the process of acquisition of knowledge and attitudes from important others, such as parents, teachers, peers and media figures. With regard to young children, it would be expected that their expression of attitudes towards alcohol will reflect this latter process – 'attitudes toward [the attitude object] are now chiefly determined not by contact with [the attitude object], but by contact with the prevalent attitude towards [the attitude object]' (Horowitz, 1947: 517).

Concerning the structure of attitudes, one school of thought (Katz and Stotland, 1959; Rajecki, 1982) proposes that attitudes are made up of three components: the 'cognitive' component refers to the beliefs and ideas one has acquired about the attitude object; the 'affective' component is the emotional feelings one has towards the attitude object; and finally the 'behavioural' component refers to one's action tendencies with regard to the attitude object. However, an alternative to this approach is described by Brigham (1991), who has suggested that attitudes can be defined as 'schemas', which usually include affect, which are used to evaluate objects. A schema or cognitive structure represents a way in which people organize their social knowledge and has been defined as: 'an organised pattern of thought or action that an individual develops to make sense of some aspect of one's experience' (Shaffer, 1989: 59). Thus, a person's schema will determine how he/she categorizes or evaluates an object.

There are four functions that attitudes are generally perceived to perform (Smith, Bruner and White, 1956; Katz, 1960). The first of these is 'understanding', in which the attitude serves to construct the world in a way that makes sense to us. The second is the 'social adjustment' function, in which the expression of certain attitudes can be understood in terms of the individual's relationship with significant others and the attitudes expressed by these significant others. The third function is that of 'ego defence'. Attitudes in this category serve to protect individuals from acknowledging uncomplimentary truths about themselves. Finally, there is the function of 'expressing values'. In these instances attitudes are seen to be expressing a person's underlying or central values. The function of an attitude can be related to attitude change. For example, an attitude that fulfils an understanding function may be changed more effectively by a strategy that employs information-based techniques. If an attitude performs a social adjustment function, then attempts to understand an attitude change should focus on the individual's changing relationships with significant others and the attitudes of those significant others, i.e. the altered social context.

Finally, Kelman (1958) has suggested three examples of social influence which may underlie the expression of a certain attitude: compliance (an external acceptance of an attitude without internal acceptance of it); identification (an acceptance of another's attitude because of an attachment to that other); and internalization (an internal acceptance of an attitude).

By applying these factors to the scores of the children in the current task, one can extrapolate an overall pattern of attitude development. The following discussion deals first of all with the general age differences in attitudes towards drinkers, and then goes on to consider the differences in attitudes between the male and female subjects and their attitudinal differences in relation to the gender of the drinker.

Despite the relatively low consistency levels recorded for the attitudes of the youngest age group, their overall scores revealed a small but nevertheless significant negative attitude towards adult drinkers. These scores would appear to reflect the acquisition of a rudimentary schema for alcohol that is being developed on the basis of observation and indirect social learning from those social role models that are salient for the child's affective and social requirements. At this early stage this role is typically filled by the parents. The structure of the schemas is primarily cognitive, with the evaluation of alcohol containing little personal affect at this time. This is illustrated by the types of responses made by these children when questioned directly about what they knew about alcohol (see Chapter 7), e.g. 'these kinds of drinks are usually drunk by grown ups', 'they make you drunk', 'my daddy drinks those kinds of things'. These mainly factual responses tend not to convey a sense of judgement or of strong internalized feelings of what is right or wrong (although the slightly negative overall scores suggest that some children have incorporated into their schemas some negative overtones associated with alcohol). Nor do children believe that the contents of their schemas reflect hard-and-fast rules. At this stage, the function of the schema is primarily one of understanding and therefore may be susceptible to modification through a change in the type of information received.

As age increases, so children's cognitive capacity and opportunities for elaboration of the schema increase. The children's schemas for alcohol are becoming more elaborate and are broadening to include an affective component which is being learned from their social role models. This is reflected in the age-related increase in the negativity of the attitudes. Again, this can also be seen in their statements regarding alcohol (see Chapter 7): e.g. 'drinking is bad' 'that man is drinking alcohol' therefore 'that man is bad'. The 'rules' of the schemas are now applied more rigidly. This adherence to the rules of such simplified or stereotypical schemas appears to function as a necessary basis for early understanding (Martin and Halverson, 1983), from which the formation of more comprehensive and flexible schemas can then be developed. The function of the attitude now becomes one of social adjustment, and for most of the young children in this group, the rewarding identification with attitudes of conventional authority figures is the key factor. However, for some of the older children, the attitude may reflect a more calculated compliance with the socially 'desirable' responses represented by the experimenter (Aitken, 1978).

The period between the ages of ten and fourteen years reveals a transitional stage during which the steady increase in negativity towards alcohol gradually declines and then reverses (Aitken, 1978). It is during this period that children are also likely to report an increase in their consumption of alcohol (May, 1991), and therefore a 'behavioural' component assumes a new relevance in the context of the increasing elaboration of the schema. Attitudes that have been formed on the basis of direct interaction with the attitude object are likely to show a greater consistency with behaviour than attitudes formed in more indirect ways (Fazio and Zanna, 1981). With regard to cognitive maturation, the previously rigid application of the 'rules' of the schema becomes more flexible, and children are more able to moderate their evaluations. Relationships with peers also become more important at this stage, although not to the exclusion of

(Kandel and Lesser, 1972; Brook and Brook. 1988), nor necessarily in opposition to (Margulies, Kessler and Kandel, 1977), parental influence. The finding that much of the early drinking that is done by teenagers takes place under the supervision and approval of their parents has been consistently confirmed by survey data (Aitken, 1978; Plant, Peck and Samuel, 1985; Marsh, Dobbs and White, 1986; Bagnall, 1988). Thus the reversal in attitudes towards drinking cannot simply be understood in terms of a change from identification with adults to rebellious identification with peers. The gradual shift to a more positive attitude can be understood, however, in terms of an expanding network of influential social relationships and a changing perspective of the social self from that of a child to that of a potential adult and therefore a potential drinker. Both the adolescent and those that socially influence him/her alter their perceptions of alcohol and alcohol use to fit this changing social identity. The function of the attitude is becoming one of expressing one's own values, as the young person tries to formulate his/her own set of guiding principles within this changing social context.

In the present exercise, female drinkers were judged more harshly than were male drinkers by all children. Initially this finding may appear somewhat incongruous with the increasing prevalence and social acceptance of alcohol use by women. It should be noted that recent survey evidence indicates that 89 per cent of women in Britain consume alcohol, even if only in small amounts (Foster, Wilmot and Dobbs, 1990). However, it may be that such 'politically correct' messages are not so evident within the home environment. Moreover, if one considers that in most drinking cultures men still remain the more frequent and more heavy drinkers (Dight, 1976; Wilson, 1980; Goddard, 1991) and are relatively more likely to experience alcohol-related problems (Plant, 1990; Plant and Plant, 1992), then such attitudes are less surprising. That alcohol consumption is primarily a male prerogative is a concept that is continually reinforced in British culture. In a study of parental attitudes towards teenage drinkers, Hawker (1978) found that parental approval of drinking did not differ with respect to the sex of the child. Even so, studies have consistently shown that boys tend to report lower ages than girls for occasion of first drink (Aitken, 1978; Davies and Stacey, 1972; Plant, Peck and Samuel, 1985; Bagnall, 1988), and that fathers are commonly the providers of the first drink (Aitken, 1978; Casswell *et al.*, 1983). Moreover, a recent survey has shown that as a group married women with dependent children have one of the lowest levels of alcohol consumption (Foster, Wilmot and Dobbs, 1990). It is possible that such behaviours might implicitly influence young children's early attitudes to female drinking. Additional evidence that young children's schemas concerning alcohol use incorporate these traditional learned sex differences comes from this study and others which show that children interpret the social norms for drinking as characteristically more male than female (Penrose, 1978; Greenberg, Zucker and Noll, 1985; Noll, Zucker and Greenberg, 1990), and attribute significantly greater liking of alcohol to men than to women (Jahoda and Cramond, 1972; Spiegler, 1983; Fossey, 1993).

The results from the current study also revealed that female subjects judged both women drinkers and women smokers (see Chapter 8 in relation to attitudes towards smoking), significantly more harshly than did the male subjects. The popular belief that girls are more 'social' than boys is commonly refuted by scientific evidence. Girls and boys are equally sensitive to social reinforcement and equally adept at learning from social role models. Also, the majority of studies reveal an absence of sex differences in children's conformity (Maccoby and Jacklin, 1974).

Martin and Halverson (1981, 1983) have proposed that young children's comprehension of gender and gender-roles can be understood in terms of the development of cognitive schemas for gender-appropriate behaviour. By the age of two or three years, children are aware of their own genders and are able to organize other people into two corresponding categories: own sex and other sex. At around five to six years the idea that gender is permanent is understood. At this stage information concerning their own gender-appropriate behaviour becomes more salient to children (Ruble, Balaban and Cooper, 1981) and this leads to the development of more elaborate gender schemas. Furthermore, a study by Fagot (1985) has shown that while boys were more sensitive to reinforcements about gender-role behaviour from other boys, girls were more sensitive to reinforcements from teachers and other girls.

What appears to be happening with the girls in this study is that they are acquiring and developing a schema about their own gender through social role models, which in turn reinforces the belief that alcohol consumption is not only an activity to be frowned upon but also that it is a 'non-feminine' activity, thus shaping the attitude. Thus, because women are more likely than men to drink wine (Foster, Wilmot and Dobbs, 1990), it is possible that girls' greater disapproval of drinking in general can then be targeted towards this more saliently feminine activity. This is not to say that boys do not also learn about female-appropriate behaviours (as is illustrated above by the more negative attitudes towards women drinkers displayed by both girls and boys), but that information regarding one's own sex will be more salient. As stated previously, this oversimplification or stereotyping of behaviour appears to be a necessary process in the eventual development of more comprehensive and flexible schemas (Martin and Halverson, 1983).

The above interpretation of the findings ties in closely with the integrative model of moral development and socialization formulated by Garbarino and Bronfenbrenner (1976). This model takes into account the influences of both developmental and social factors in the process of moral socialization. Previous theories have tended to concentrate on either one (Kohlberg, 1969) or the other (Bronfenbrenner, 1962) respectively. Thus such a model can adequately account for the fact that the development of attitudes does not proceed at a uniform rate for all children. It can also explain why individual children's attitudes towards various attitude objects do not necessarily develop at the same rates. In the present study, the former can be seen simply in the variation and similarity of responses for children within and between each age group. The significant variations in attitudes between the different socio-economic status, sex and verbal fluency groups also lend weight to this. The latter point is illustrated by the attitude scores on the smoking items (see Chapter 8). Although similar attitude trends can be seen in both the drinking and smoking scores, the negativity towards smoking is already more clearly established in the youngest age group. The source and content of health messages concerning alcohol are varied and often conflicting. In contrast, messages concerning smoking are less confused and therefore more coherent.

Finally, young children's attitudes towards alcohol have changed surprisingly little during the past twenty years. Only two significant differences between the two studies emerged: in the current sample older children were slightly less negative towards male drinkers; and female drinkers were judged more negatively by girls than by boys only in the current sample. These findings imply that the social messages concerning alcohol which are effectively transmitted to children have, on the whole, remained relatively stable over this period, with few exceptions. This stability is remarkable since, as already stated, alcohol consumption in the United Kingdom has risen markedly since the 1970s.

The finding that girls were more condemnatory than boys of women drinkers, in the present sample only, was contrary to expectations, in light of recent increases in the number of women now consuming alcohol, and more generally in view of the increasing value imposed by society on the issue of sexual equality. Unfortunately, it is not possible to compare with any great accuracy these present-day attitudes to those of children twenty years ago, as 'drinking wine' was not included as an item in Jahoda and Cramond's study. As speculated previously, it is possible that young girls are simply more likely to see women drinking wine than either beer or whisky. The proliferation of the mass media and their role in the communication of socio-cultural values has also provided children with an additional source of information. The now ubiquitous image of the attractive 'macho' drinker portrayed in the media (Finn and Strickland, 1982) may thus in part account for the small decrease in negativity towards male drinkers. It may also be the case that while the media are perpetuating a more positive image of the male drinker, they are at the same time endorsing an unrepresentative image of the female drinker. For example, the female characters Sue Ellen in the soap opera *Dallas* and Cagney in the detective series *Cagney and Lacey* are both portrayed as problem drinkers. That is not to say that the media are responsible for the attitudes, but rather that it may serve to reinforce children's early perceptions.

THE PERCEIVED LIKES AND DISLIKES TASK

Drinking habits have changed markedly since the time of Jahoda and Cramond's study. The level of per capita consumption in the United Kingdom reached a post-war peak in 1979. Since then, despite a slight decline, this level has been slowly drifting upwards, although it still remains lower than in 1979. Beer remains the most commonly consumed alcoholic drink in the UK, although the popularity of wine has increased considerably over the past thirty years. Spirit consumption has increased more slowly and more erratically over the years and remains at a considerably lower level than that for other alcoholic drinks. Currently over 90 per cent of British adults drink alcohol at least occasionally: younger adults drink more than older adults; men drink more frequently and more heavily than women (Goddard and Ikin, 1988). However, there is now a tendency for more British women (89 per cent) to consume alcohol, if only in small amounts (Foster, Wilmot and Dobbs, 1990). It was predicted that the data collected in the present investigation, when compared with Jahoda and Cramond's earlier study, might reflect these changes.

The 'Perceived Likes and Dislikes' task in Jahoda and Cramond's report was designed to examine children's understanding of social norms such as these above relating to drinking behaviour. That is, to discover children's perceptions of what constitutes 'normal' alcohol-related behaviour in three social groups, namely men, women and children. Again, the inappropriateness of direct verbal questioning necessitated an indirect approach. For this reason, the method of inquiry adopted was based upon eliciting children's perceptions of how much men, women and children liked or disliked certain activities related to drinking alcohol. These activities were as follows: drinking beer; drinking whisky; going to the pub (public bar); and being drunk. On the basis of their preference attributions it would then be possible to construe basic images of the social norms held by these subjects.

Jahoda and Cramond found that children attributed dislike of all four alcohol-related activities to women and children, but not to men. Only when the role in question was male did children's scores indicate a perceived liking, and even then, only in relation to beer drinking. In general, boys gave higher liking scores than girls irrespective of the social group under consideration. Furthermore, perceived liking scores tended to decrease as age of subject rose.

In accordance with the approach employed by Jahoda and Cramond, in the present exercise this task was carried out over two sessions, each of which consisted of three trials. In the first session a pre-recorded tape of a list of non-alcohol-related activities suitable for male and female adults and children was played to the subjects. On the first trial, a child toy doll (representing a child of the same sex as the subject) was placed in front of the child. On hearing each activity on the list, the subject was required to decide how much this 'child' would like or dislike doing the activity according to the following four categories: 'Like very much'; ' Like a little'; 'Do not like a little'; and 'Do not like at all'. The second and third trials were conducted in the same manner, using an adult male doll and an adult female doll in order to represent men and women respectively. All responses were registered on a computer. The second session was conducted in a similar way, the only difference being that the lists now contained the following alcohol-related activities: drinking beer; drinking whisky; drinking wine; going to a public bar; and finally, being drunk. Again, the item 'drinking wine' was a new addition to the task. A more comprehensive description of the methodology of this exercise is given in Chapter 3.

Results

For the purpose of comparing the current results with those found by Jahoda and Cramond, these scores were again computed according to the procedures adopted by those authors. As before, during the 'Judgement of Photographs' task, consistency of responses on this task was measured by means of the repeated items. Four items/activities were repeated in both of the sessions, resulting in a total of eight pairs of repeated items for each of the three trials. Consistency was thus defined as six of the eight possible pairs falling on the same side of the like/dislike division. Not surprisingly, subjects' responses to children's likes/dislikes showed the highest consistency overall, at 93 per cent. When the role was that of women, consistency was 86.8 per cent, while for men the figure was 85.9 per cent. Crosstabulations of consistency scores by age revealed a significant age effect for women only ($X^2 = 13.96$; 6df; $p < 0.03$), with the youngest age group reporting more inconsistent responses when the role involved was the adult woman. This would seem to support the contention that male roles are more clearly delineated than those of females.

Scores for the main task were derived by assigning arbitrary scores of 1 to 4 to the response categories 'Do not like at all', 'Do not like a little', 'Like a little' and 'Like a lot' respectively. Mean scores were then calculated for the pooled 'food' items and for each of the 'alcohol-related' and 'smoking-related' items. The remaining buffer items were ignored. Mean scores were them multiplied by 10 in order to produce rounded whole numbers, producing in turn a range of possible scores from 10 (extreme dislike) to 40 (maximum liking) with a neutral point of 25.

In Jahoda and Cramond's study, the analysis of the 'food' items within the lists of activities was included as a control measure to ensure that children were performing this task correctly. These authors proposed that if differences in children's perceptions for liking food occurred between the three roles, then this would invalidate their subsequent scores for the main items consisting of the alcohol-related activities. The reasoning behind this was that if children differentiated between preferences for food for these roles, this would imply that their perceptions were based upon individuals, e.g. themselves or their parents, for, as these authors argued, there are no recognized social role norms relating to food preferences. In the current study, multivariate analysis of the data relating to the food items revealed no significant main effects in terms of between-subject groups but a significant effect in terms of the roles was revealed.

However, in contrast to Jahoda and Cramond, it is argued that this does not necessarily invalidate the remaining data. As can be seen in the description of items used in this task (shown in Appendix 2), these lists contained a variety of such items referring to various vegetables, non-alcoholic drinks, sweets, etc. It is clear that these comprise a number of items that are more likely or less likely to be liked/disliked by children. In addition, women/mothers may commonly be seen to encourage other family members to eat certain foodstuffs which their family or indeed they themselves do not particularly enjoy. Finally, men in general are commonly considered to have more indiscriminate appetites. These are evidently examples of what may be perceived to constitute 'normative' eating behaviours, and for this reason analysis of the remaining data was continued. Thus, the mean scores for each of the alcohol-related items are shown in Table 5.6.

Overall, children were perceived to dislike all five alcohol-related activities. Women were perceived as liking only drinking wine, while men were perceived as liking all alcohol-related items with the exception of 'being drunk'. In fact, a dislike of 'being drunk' was attributed to all three roles/identities (i.e. to men, women and children). However, men were perceived as disliking this activity significantly less than women and children, who were perceived as disliking this activity equally.

Separate multivariate analyses of variance were carried out for all five alcohol-related activities, in order to establish what factors, if any, might have significantly influenced children's perceptions. These results are shown in Tables 5.7–5.11. Again, for the purpose of minimizing the presentation of this information, only those interaction effects which were significant are shown.

Perceptions of likes/dislikes for the item 'drinking beer' differed significantly according to the sex of subjects, with girls perceiving greater dislike than boys of beer drinking, regardless of the social identity of the drinker (i.e. whether the person was a man, woman or child). However, when the identity of the drinker was taken into account, it was found that the female subjects attributed greater dislike of drinking beer to girls than did the male subjects to boys. (Note that when the trial relating to children's preferences was conducted, the female subjects were presented with a female doll only, while the male subjects were presented with a male doll only.) Similarly, when the role was again that of a child, older subjects attributed greater dislike of this activity to children than did the younger subjects, as did middle-class subjects in comparison to

Table 5.6 Mean perception scores by age of subject

	Age							
	5–6 yrs		7–8 yrs		9–10 yrs		5–10 yrs	
	Mean	*SD*	*Mean*	*SD*	*Mean*	*SD*	*Mean*	*SD*
Beer								
Child	21.22	12.04	17.12	10.83	13.67	7.77	17.31	10.77
Woman	18.58	10.22	20.26	11.16	18.80	9.51	19.23	10.31
Man	32.70	10.41	34.10	9.00	34.20	7.93	33.68	9.15
Whisky								
Child	18.31	11.48	15.83	9.31	13.00	6.31	15.70	9.47
Woman	22.50	11.91	23.21	11.05	23.27	10.08	23.00	10.99
Man	29.19	11.62	29.94	9.48	30.00	9.62	29.71	10.23
Wine								
Child	22.57	13.25	19.62	11.22	16.53	9.51	19.56	11.63
Woman	27.70	12.88	30.00	11.95	28.13	10.87	28.63	11.91
Man	30.00	12.39	31.15	10.81	29.33	10.95	30.18	11.37
Pub								
Child	24.05	13.34	18.33	11.67	16.93	11.03	19.74	12.37
Woman	24.05	13.94	21.67	12.42	21.60	10.14	22.42	12.26
Man	33.51	11.39	33.08	11.09	34.40	9.04	33.66	10.53
Drunk								
Child	15.54	10.36	12.56	7.46	12.13	6.64	13.39	8.38
Woman	15.54	9.81	13.08	7.44	13.07	7.88	13.88	8.46
Man	20.00	12.82	21.54	13.00	20.00	12.41	20.53	12.71

Scores range from 10 (maximum dislike) to 40 (maximum liking).

working-class subjects. Finally, the identity of the drinker significantly affected performance overall, with children generally attributing greater liking of beer to men, in contrast to women and children who were perceived to dislike this activity.

Similarly, the identity of the drinker also had a significant impact on liking scores for the item 'drinking whisky'. Children were perceived as disliking whisky more than women, and men were perceived as liking whisky more than both women and children. Again, there were significant interactions in terms of the different age groups and gender groups. In both cases older children and girls perceived greater dislike of drinking whisky among similar children than did their respective counterparts. However, there were no corresponding

Table 5.7 Attributions of likes/dislikes of 'drinking beer'

	SS	DF	MS	F	SIG (P)
Between subjects					
Within cells	19686.67	145	135.77		
Constant	348763.62	1	348763.62	2568.78	0.000
Age (A)	524.66	2	262.33	1.93	NS
Sex (B)	858.55	1	858.55	6.32	0.013
Ses. (C)	120.78	1	120.78	< 1	NS
City (D)	0.01	1	0.01	< 1	NS
Religion (E)	214.42	1	214.42	1.58	NS
BPVS (F)	332.29	1	332.29	2.45	NS
Within subjects					
Within cells	17390.00	290	59.97		
Drinker identity (G)	34785.43	2	17392.71	290.05	0.000
A * G	1935.90	4	483.97	8.07	0.000
B * G	1519.30	2	759.65	12.67	0.000
C * G	415.35	2	207.68	3.46	0.033

Table 5.8 Attributions of likes/dislikes of 'drinking whisky'

	SS	DF	MS	F	SIG (P)
Between subjects					
Within cells	25659.17	145	176.96		
Constant	333925.77	1	333925.77	1887.02	0.000
Age (A)	193.87	2	96.94	< 1	NS
Sex (B)	134.58	1	134.58	< 1	NS
Ses. (C)	50.93	1	50.93	< 1	NS
City (D)	146.41	1	146.41	< 1	NS
Religion (E)	23.09	1	23.09	< 1	NS
BPVS (F)	28.29	1	28.29	< 1	NS
Within subjects					
Within cells	17435.00	290	60.12		
Drinker identity (G)	21037.18	2	10518.59	174.96	0.000
A * G	958.58	4	239.64	3.99	0.004
B * G	1521.30	2	760.64	12.65	0.000

differences in terms of social class on this occasion. These results are shown in Table 5.8.

In relation to the third specific type of alcoholic drink, men and

Table 5.9 Attributions of likes/dislikes of 'drinking wine'

	SS	DF	MS	F	SIG (P)
Between subjects					
Within cells	27316.11	145	188.39		
Constant	438242.14	1	438242.14	2326.29	0.000
Age (A)	719.03	2	359.52	1.91	NS
Sex (B)	607.93	1	607.93	3.23	NS
Ses. (C)	1247.72	1	1247.72	6.62	0.011
City (D)	406.56	1	406.56	2.16	NS
Religion (E)	16.29	1	16.29	< 1	NS
BPVS (F)	25.44	1	25.44	< 1	NS
Within subjects					
Within cells	29455.56	290	101.57		
Drinker identity (G)	14210.33	2	7105.16	69.95	0.000
A * G	1015.18	4	253.80	2.50	0.043
D * G	621.26	2	310.63	3.06	0.048

women were both perceived to enjoy drinking wine, in contrast to children who were again perceived to dislike this activity (see Table 5.9). In particular, the middle-class children perceived drinking wine to be an activity that was generally enjoyed more so than did the working-class children. Interaction effects occurred again when the identity of the drinker was that of a child. Older children and children from Edinburgh were more likely than younger subjects and those from Birmingham respectively to attribute to children a dislike of wine.

Table 5.10 refers to subjects' perceptions of likes/dislikes of going to a public bar. Men were more likely to be perceived as liking this activity than were women and children, both of whom were perceived to dislike this activity. Both older children and girls perceived a greater general dislike of this activity than did younger subjects and boys, irrespective of social identity, although these trends were particularly apparent when the role under consideration was that of the child. Edinburgh subjects and those from Birmingham differed in their perceived likes/dislikes for all three roles. The former subjects attributed greater dislike of this activity than the latter subjects when the roles were those of the child and the woman, but perceived less dislike when the role was that of the man.

In relation to the final item 'being drunk', age and sex of subject made no difference to the scores. That is, subjects of all ages and both sexes attributed similar levels of dislike in relation to all roles.

Table 5.10 Attributions of likes/dislikes of 'going to the pub'

	SS	DF	MS	F	SIG (P)
Between subjects					
Within cells	30254.44	145	208.65		
Constant	406799.94	1	406799.94	1949.66	0.000
Age (A)	1319.44	2	659.72	3.16	0.045
Sex (B)	1371.39	1	1371.39	6.57	0.011
Ses. (C)	27.80	1	27.80	< 1	NS
City (D)	193.73	1	193.73	< 1	NS
Religion (E)	87.99	1	87.99	< 1	NS
BPVS (F)	394.75	1	394.75	1.89	NS
Within subjects					
Within cells	25678.89	290	88.55		
Drinker identity (G)	23168.14	2	11584.07	130.82	0.000
A * G	1148.87	4	287.22	3.24	0.013
B * G	739.72	2	369.86	4.18	0.016
D * G	2425.17	2	1212.59	13.69	0.000

Table 5.11 Attributions of likes/dislikes of 'being drunk'

	SS	DF	MS	F	SIG (P)
Between subjects					
Within cells	20209.44	145	139.38		
Constant	158034.81	1	158034.81	1133.88	0.000
Age (A)	552.68	2	276.34	1.98	NS
Sex (B)	454.26	1	454.26	3.26	NS
Ses. (C)	1412.46	1	1412.46	10.13	0.002
City (D)	113.17	1	113.17	< 1	NS
Religion (E)	47.78	1	47.78	< 1	NS
BPVS (F)	1110.60	1	1110.60	7.97	0.005
Within subjects					
Within cells	18778.89	290	64.75		
Drinker identity (G)	6632.04	2	3316.02	51.21	0.000
E * G	534.35	2	267.18	4.13	0.017

However, middle-class children gave higher disliking scores for 'being drunk' than did working-class children. So too did those children scoring higher on the British Picture Vocabulary Scale when compared with low scorers. In addition, social identity also signifi-cantly influenced perceptions, with men generally perceived to dislike being drunk less than women and children. Finally, when the role was that of the child, subjects attending Roman Catholic schools attribu-ted greater dislike of this activity to children than did those subjects attending non-denominational schools.

Discussion

The results from this task confirm that from an early age, children are developing conceptions about normative drinking behaviour. Overall, children were perceived to dislike all five alcohol-related activities. With the exception of the item 'drinking wine', both boys and girls perceived that women generally disliked alcohol. Subjects also perceived that women disliked being drunk as much as children did. Men were perceived as liking all alcohol-related activities with the exception of 'being drunk'.

There were no differences in relation to perceived adult prefer-ences between the three subject age groups, indicating that, at least in relation to adult behaviour, by the age of five and a half years children have already acquired the relevant 'social category knowl-edge' (Higgins, Feldman and Ruble, 1980) necessary to establish drinking norms for these role categories. However, several subject-group differences did emerge when the child role was considered. Female subjects generally perceived a greater dislike of alcohol-related activities for girls, than did male subjects for boys. In addition, children's perceived dislike of alcohol-related activities increased with rising age of subject (although it is important to stress that the mean scores of even the youngest children fell into the 'dislike' category).

Several other subject differences also emerged for the individual drinking activities. These factors included verbal intelligence, social class, city and religious affiliation differences. With regard to these between-subject trends there are two possible explanations for why they should occur. One is associated with the types strategies which children make use of when making social judgements. The other refers to the type of knowledge they possess which forms the basis for making these judgements.

As children grow older and their cognitive development pro-gresses, their repertoire for making social judgements also becomes more elaborate. The process of 'social reference' (Higgins, Feldman and Ruble, 1980) refers to the technique of choosing a more representative category member with which to judge the normality of another category member's behaviour over one that is simply more salient. For example, it has been suggested that younger children generally tend to refer to their parents when asked to make judgements concerning adult preferences, whereas older children and adults are more likely to choose popular media figures. Taking this into account with subjects' perceptions of children's preferences in the current exercise, it may be that the older children have learnt to reject the more salient member of the category (i.e. themselves) in favour of a more representative/typical category member. If this were the case in this sample, then one might assume that the like/dislike perceptions of the older children would be more consistent and more accurate. However, an alternative strategy may have been an 'assumed similarity' on the part of the children, between their own preferences and those of their peers. In the study by Higgins, Feldman and Ruble (1980), three groups of subjects – four to five year olds, eight to nine year olds, and undergraduates – were required to select from a variety of objects the one which they themselves would prefer. On subsequent trials, these same subjects were then required to select the object which they felt was most likely to be preferred by their peers and, again, the object they felt would be most preferred by non-peers. Higgins and his colleagues found that subjects within each age group would select their own preference for peers, significantly more often than they would select their own preference for non-peers. Furthermore, within each age group, the consensus in selecting the most preferred item for each target group was significantly greater than by chance.

The second possible explanation for the between-subject differences in the results lies in both the extent of information and the nature of the information which these subjects possess. That is, children may be differentially exposed to opportunities for various aspects of social learning which will expand and shape their schemas for alcohol. Using the age of subject differences as an illustration of this, it may be that due to their age-related increase in exposure to such opportunities, the older subjects have been able to reinforce the fact that alcoholic drinks are not appropriate for children but are the exclusive domain of adults.

If one considers the attitudes of these same children towards adult drinking in general, discussed in the first half of this chapter, it can be seen that the younger subjects were less likely than those who are older to have formed firm attitudes towards alcohol consumption. However, attitudes towards adult drinking became increasingly negative as the children grew older. As was stressed previously, although the perceived dislike among children for alcohol-related activities increased with age of subject, the perceptions of the youngest subjects, while less consistent overall, were, however, already negative. Thus, it appears likely that neither increasing judgement ability nor accuracy *per se* are wholly responsible for the age-related changes in norm perceptions, but rather that the latter are also likely to be subject to the increasing, and increasingly negative, content of children's schemas for alcohol in relation to their relevant 'social category knowledge'. Such a theory is confirmed by the children's scores for the smoking preference perceptions (see Chapter 8). In relation to the smoking items, there were no significant differences in scores with regard to age when the role was that of the child. The youngest children had already established that children as a group do not like smoking either cigarettes or a pipe.

An explanation in terms of type and extent of knowledge would also be consistent with the other between-subject differences such as religion, city and sex of subject, as it is unlikely that these differences would be the result of clear-cut corresponding differences in social judgement strategies. Main effects for sex of subject when the role was that of the child showed a sex-stereotyped pattern. When the role was that of the child, boys and girls differed significantly in their perceptions of dislike. Girls attributed greater dislike of alcohol-related activities for girls as a group, than did boys for boys as a group. Unfortunately it was not possible to perform a cross-sex comparison to ascertain whether female subjects perceived boys' likes/dislikes of alcohol-related activities to the same extent as the male subjects did and vice versa, or whether the female subjects do believe that girls as a group do in fact dislike such activities more than boys. Other studies that have incorporated a cross-sex comparison have generally found no such sex differences (Penrose, 1978; Greenberg, Zucker and Noll, 1985; Zucker, Fitzgerald and Noll, 1991). However, in the first part of this chapter it was demonstrated that the female subjects did display more negative attitudes than did the male subjects towards adult female drinkers.

The fact that social class exhibited a main effect on scores relating to drinking wine was interesting. Middle-class subjects gave significantly higher liking scores than working-class subjects regardless of role, suggesting that wine fulfils a markedly different function as perceived by these two groups of subjects. Recent OPCS data shows that non-manual-working men, and non-manual-working women particularly, are more likely to be drinkers than are manual workers

(Foster, Wilmot and Dobbs, 1990). Moreover, although Foster and her colleagues did not differentiate between the drink preferences of these two social groups, the data which do exist confirm that the type of alcoholic drink most often consumed by women generally is wine. Therefore it might be construed that due to the female drinkers, middle-class families are more likely than working-class families to drink wine, a trend more recently supported by Loretto (personal communication) in relation to drinking habits in young people.

The two study areas, Birmingham in the West Midlands and Edinburgh in the Lothian region, have a considerably different mix of ethnic populations. The West Midlands has one of the highest concentrations of ethnic minorities outside of the south-east of England, at 6.8 per cent or around 1 in 15 of the population. In contrast, only 1.1 per cent of the population of Scotland as a whole is made up of ethnic minority races. In both areas, the majority of the ethnic population is made up of peoples from India/Pakistan and Bangladesh who, for religious reasons, may be more likely to abstain from alcohol consumption. In addition, percentages of household expenditure on alcohol and tobacco products vary between the two areas. The figure for the West Midlands is 6.1 per cent with the higher figure of 7.3 per cent for Scotland as a whole. For these reasons, it might reasonably be predicted that the Birmingham half of the sample would likewise display lower liking scores for drinking alcohol than those from Edinburgh. However, this was not the case. In fact, if anything, subjects from Edinburgh tended to attribute greater dislike of certain alcohol-related activities, when significant differences between the two study areas were found.

Although the study group as a whole demonstrated very high dislike scores in relation to the item 'being drunk' as expected, some subject groups attributed greater dislike than others. Both middle-class children and those who scored higher on the British Picture Vocabulary Scale gave significantly greater disliking scores for this item irrespective of the identity of the drinker. However, Roman Catholic children perceived greater dislike of 'being drunk' than did children attending non-denominational schools only in relation to children. In contrast, preliminary data from Loretto (personal communication) suggests that Northern Irish Roman Catholic teenagers may be less disapproving of drunkenness than their Protestant counterparts.

Finally, in comparison with Jahoda and Cramond's findings, the present results suggest that children's perceptions of cultural norms associated with drinking habits have changed somewhat over the past twenty years. Alcohol was perceived as being more enjoyed by men and less disliked by women and children by the children in the present study than by the children in Jahoda and Cramond's study. Nevertheless, in view of national trends, these current perceptions still appear to vastly under-represent actual adult preferences. The present sample, however, still displayed a rather stereotyped image of women in relation to alcohol-related activities. Unfortunately, Jahoda and Cramond did not report on differences relating to social class, city, etc., thus preventing the possibility of further comparisons.

As stated previously, Martin and Halverson (1981, 1983) have proposed that children's comprehension of gender and gender roles can be understood in terms of their development of cognitive schemas for gender-appropriate behaviour. By the age of five or six years, information about their own gender becomes more salient to children (Ruble, Balaban and Cooper, 1981), and by social learning from prominent role models this leads to the formation of more elaborate gender schemas. Thus, the perceptions of the boys and girls in this study can be understood in terms of their acquisition of relevant social category knowledge via social learning from significant role models, and therefore, in accordance with Borgida, Locksley and Brekke (1981), such social stereotypes can be viewed 'as products of normal everyday cognitive processes of social categorisation, social inference, and social judgement'.

6 Children's familiarity with the physical manifestations of drunkenness and their expectations of alcohol

THE DRUNKENNESS FILMS TASK

When children are asked about the consequences of drinking alcoholic beverages, they invariably refer to the acute effects of intoxication and, in particular, the state of being drunk. Moreover, very rarely do they qualify drunkenness in terms of quantity of alcohol consumed (Casswell *et al.*, 1983). However, although children appear to be familiar with the verbal label 'drunk' from an early stage, it does not necessarily follow that they have a full grasp of the concept of drunkenness, i.e. that they are familiar with the repertoire of the possible social and behavioural implications of alcohol consumption.

In their study, Jahoda and Cramond incorporated into their test battery a task designed to examine the stage at which young children are able to infer drunkenness from a person's behaviour. Salient behavioural indicators of the drunken state include both verbal cues, e.g. slurred speech, and non-verbal cues, e.g. loss of control over bodily movement. As neither of these can be conveyed by still photographs, Jahoda and Cramond devised a short film consisting in brief of a man drinking in a public bar and staggering drunkenly down the street. The film itself was made up of four consecutive parts, which were shown to the children in reverse chronological order – i.e. they would see the behavioural consequences of excessive drinking before they saw the cause behind the behaviour.

Due to insufficient resources, these authors were unable to add a sound track to the film, so the children were forced to rely on non-verbal cues alone. However, in spite of receiving fewer cues than would be expected in a real 'encounter', the children in Jahoda and Cramond's study were extremely successful at identifying drunkenness purely in terms of physical characteristics. Just over 94 per cent of the total sample recognized that the actor was exhibiting drunken behaviour after observing only the final section of the film. As might be expected, the youngest children tended to require more parts of the film to be shown. Nevertheless, not even one child required the entire film to be shown in order to recognize the drunkenness theme. Due to the high success rate exhibited by these children, Jahoda and Cramond conducted the same test on a small group of four-year-old children ($n = 14$). Three children (21.4 per cent) were successful following only the final section of the film, and only two children (14.3 per cent) failed to understand the drunkenness theme following presentation of the entire film.

Further questionning of the older main sample during the presentation of the film revealed that 95 per cent of the children had observed drunkenness on a first-hand basis. Of this group, the majority (70.3 per cent) reported having seen drunks in the street. Just over 15 per cent mentioned that their experience of drunks had occurred within their home, and 14.4 per cent reported seeing drunks in a bar-room. Only 2.5 per cent of the total sample mentioned the television or cinema as the source of their experience of intoxicated people.

In the present study this task took on a similar format to that designed by Jahoda and Cramond. However, it was decided to include a version of the film featuring a female, in order to examine the possibility that the sex of the drunk person might affect children's responses. It was hypothesized that a film of an intoxicated female would evoke different responses to those elicited by that of a male drunk, in two ways: first, children would be slower to attribute drunkenness to the female because children may not readily associate drunkenness with women in general; and second, because previous evidence has indicated that children are more condemnatory of female alcohol use, children's attitudes towards the drunk woman would be more critical. More generally, it was predicted that attitudes towards the drunken characters would become increasingly hostile among older children, in accordance with their attitudes towards adult drinking.

The methods employed in the current study have been described in Chapter 3, but in brief, this task was divided into three phases, each involving the presentation of a video film designed to portray different bodily and mental states. The first phase consisted of a training film to familiarize children with the task procedure, the second was the main experimental task dealing with drunkenness, and the third was included to reduce the salience of the alcohol theme. The current study did have the facilities to add a sound track. Even so, because of the high success rate shown by Jahoda and Cramond's sample, even without sound cues, it was decided that the newly made films would be silent. Five video films were made in total, each consisting of four action sequences. The initial training film consisted of a film of a young boy going shopping with his mother for a present, the target emotion in this film being happiness; the second phase was the main experimental stage concerned with drunkenness – two separate films were made dealing with this theme, one in which the drunk character was a man, the other in which the drunk character was a woman; the third phase consisted of a film in which the character was taking part in some form of exercise, the target state being exhaustion – this too had both a male and female version. The films were constructed so that they could be played in reverse chronological order, cumulatively – i.e. the final clip of the film or section D would be shown first, followed by sections C and D, then sections BCD and finally the entire film ABCD.

Results

The rate at which subjects successfully recognized the physical manifestations of drunkenness is shown in Figure 6.1. The majority, (79 per cent), did so following only the initial presentation of section D of the film. Only eight children (3.4 per cent) failed to identify the drunkenness theme following presentation of the entire film, four of whom mentioned drinking but clearly did not understand that the person was drunk, and four of whom completely failed to understand the theme. In comparison with the subjects in Jahoda and Cramond's study, the present sample were significantly less successful following the initial presentation of the film ($X^2 = 23.383$; 1df; $p < 0.00001$).

In order to tease out possible differences in subjects' performance between (1) the male and female versions of the film and (2) the various subgroups of subjects in the sample, forward stepwise logistic regression analysis was carried out on the data, the results of which are shown in Table 6.1.

Both the sex of the intoxicated character and age of subject significantly affected performance on this task. When the drunk character was female, the two older groups were increasingly more likely than the youngest subjects to demonstrate immediate recognition. That is, the youngest children were the slowest to identity the drunkenness theme when the person in the film was the woman. This probably explains why the present sample as a whole were slower at recognition overall compared to Jahoda and Cramond's sample, as the

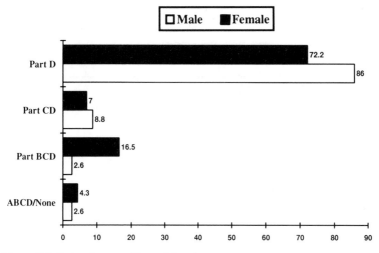

Figure 6.1 Rate of recognition of drunkenness

Table 6.1 Recognition of drunkenness (predicting the likelihood of recognizing drunkenness at once)

Parameter (reference categories in brackets)	Log odds	95% C.I. ↓	↑
Sex of drunk (male)			
Sex of drunk (2)-female	−2.6800	−4.0330	−1.3270
Age (5–6 yrs)			
Age (2) 7–8 yrs	−0.1474	−1.5430	1.2482
Age (3) 9–10 yrs	−0.0810	−1.5318	1.3698
Sex of subject (male)			
Sex of subject (2) female	−0.7844	−1.9782	0.4094
Ses. (m-c)			
Ses. (2) w-c	3.2670	1.5684	4.9656
City (Edinburgh)			
City (2) Birmingham	0.5168	−0.7974	1.8310
*Sex of drunk *age*			
Sex of drunk (2) *age (2)	2.4100	0.5292	4.2908
Sex of drunk (2) *age (3)	3.133	1.0990	5.1670
*Sex of subject *city*			
Sex (2) *city (2)	2.1580	0.5150	3.8010
*Ses. *city*			
Ses. (2) *city (2)	4.3670	−6.4270	−2.3070

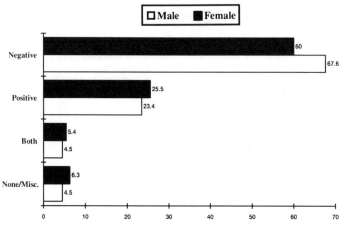

Figure 6.2 Opinions of drunk character

latter did not incorporate a 'female' version. In addition, among the female subjects in the study, those from Birmingham were significantly more likely than those from Edinburgh to identify the drunkenness theme quickly. Finally, in Edinburgh particularly, working-class subjects were more likely than middle-class subjects to be quick at recognizing drunkenness.

Children's opinions of drunk person

Taking the sample as a whole, but excluding the eight children mentioned above, just under 64 per cent ($n = 141$) expressed a negative opinion towards the drunk person. Although 24.4 per cent expressed a positive opinion, a further twelve children (5.4 per cent) felt that they did not have sufficient information to make such a judgement. Subjects' opinions with respect to the sex of the drunk character are shown in Figure 6.2.

Logistic regression analysis of these data failed to produce an adequate model. For this reason separate chi-square analyses were conducted, the results of which are shown below in Table 6.2. Children's responses to this question were divided into two categories: 'negative' and 'other'. The latter included all responses that were not negative.

Interestingly, subjects did not differ in their opinions when responses to the male film were compared with responses to the female film. Younger subjects were more likely than older subjects to

Table 6.2 Opinion of drunk character

Age	5–6 yrs	7–8 yrs	9–10 yrs	Total
Other	36	27	17	80
Negative	33	49	59	141
Total	69	76	76	221

Chi-square = 13.9338; 2df; p < 0.0009.

Ses.	m-c	w-c	Total
Other	49	31	80
Negative	61	80	141
Total	110	111	221

Chi-square = 6.6059; 1df; p < 0.0102.

City	Edinburgh	Birmingham	Total
Other	46	34	80
Negative	62	79	141
Total	108	113	221

Chi-square = 3.7384; 1df; p < 0.0532.

express an opinion that was not negative, irrespective of the sex of the intoxicated person. Similarly, subjects from Edinburgh and those from middle-class backgrounds were generally less likely than their respective counterparts to be negative towards drunks, also irrespective of the sex of the drunk character.

Drunk characters' perceived feelings

When subjects were asked how they thought the drunk person felt, just under two-thirds (65.6 per cent) of the sample gave a negative response. Just over a fifth of the sample (25.3 per cent) gave a positive response. This was only just significantly less than the proportion of children in Jahoda and Cramond's sample who thought that the drunk person 'felt good' (X^2 = 6.745; 2df; p < 0.05). These results, in terms of the sex of the intoxicated character, are shown in Figure 6.3.

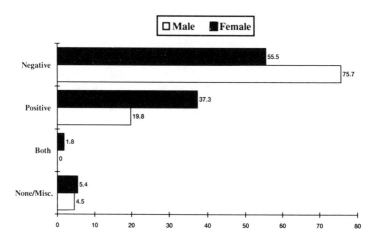

Figure 6.3 Feelings attributed to drunk person

Again, regression analysis failed to provide an adequate model so separate chi-square analyses were conducted. As before, the response categories were condensed into two distinct categories: 'negative' and 'other', i.e. all other responses. The results are shown in Table 6.3

The gender of the drunk character had a significant impact on subjects' perceptions of the drunk person's feelings. The male drunk was more likely than the female drunk to elicit negative responses. An interaction effect also occurred with this factor, with subjects from Edinburgh more likely to attribute negative feelings towards the male drunk than towards the female drunk, whereas in Birmingham, subjects appeared not to distinguish between these two film versions. Finally, among the working-class children, it was the boys who were more likely than the girls to attribute negative emotions to the drunk, irrespective of the latter's gender, while middle-class boys and girls were similar in their attributions.

Experience of drunks

Of the total sample, just under 65 per cent claimed to have previously seen a drunk person, as shown in Table 6.4. Because this was a lower figure than expected, 'sex of drunk' was retained as a factor in the following logistic regression analysis, in order to ascertain whether

Table 6.3 Perceived feelings of drunk person

Sex of drunk	Male	Female	Total
Other	27	49	76
Negative	84	61	145
Total	111	110	221

Chi-square = 10.0124; 1df; p < 0.0016.

Edinburgh*	Male D	Female D	Total		Birmingham†	Male D	Female D	Total
Other	9	27	36		Other	18	22	40
Negative	45	27	72		Negative	39	34	73
Total	54	54	108		Total	57	56	113

* Chi-square = 13.5000; 1df; p < 0.0002.
† Chi-square = 0.73367; 1df; not significant.

Middle-class*	Male D	Female D	Total		Working-class†	Male D	Female D	Total
Other	20	18	38		Other	13	25	38
Negative	33	39	72		Negative	42	31	73
Total	53	57	110		Total	55	56	111

* Chi-square = 0.46041; 1df; not significant.
† Chi-square = 5.4384; 1df; p < 0.0197.

Table 6.4 Previous sightings of drunks

	Age				
	5–6 yrs N	7–8 yrs N	9–10 yrs N	5–10 yrs N	Total %
Yes	35	48	60	143	64.7
No/dk/none	34	28	16	78	35.3
	69	76	76	221	100

'dk' represents the response 'don't know'.

Table 6.5 Experience of drunks (predicting the likelihood of having previously seen a drunk person)

Parameter (reference categories in brackets)	Log odds	95% C.I.	
		↓	↑
Ses. (m-c)			
Ses. (2) w-c	0.6323	−0.2843	1.5489
Religion (Catholic)			
Religion (2) non-den.	−0.8768	−1.7470	−0.0066
Age (5–6 yrs)			
Age (2) 7–8 yrs	0.6420	−0.1258	1.4098
Age (3) 9–10 yrs	1.5500	0.7104	2.3896
City (Edinburgh)			
City (2) Birmingham	−1.5750	−2.2596	−0.8904
*Ses. * Religion*			
Ses. (2) *Religion (2)	1.3900	0.0694	2.7106

or not children presented with the female version of the film were giving responses in terms of drunk women rather than in terms of drunk people generally. However, as can be seen in Table 6.5, the lack of significant effect for 'sex of drunk' would indicate that this was not the case.

In relation to between-subject differences, the oldest subjects were more likely than younger children to have seen a drunk person, not surprisingly. In contrast, children from Birmingham were less likely than children from Edinburgh to say that they had seen an intoxicated person. Finally with regard to religion, both Catholic and non-denominational working-class subjects were more likely than

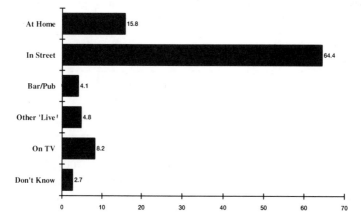

Figure 6.4 Location of sightings

middle-class subjects to state that they had seen a drunk person, although, this effect was stronger in relation to non-denominational schoolchildren.

Figure 6.4 shows the location of previous sightings of drunks reported by the subjects. Having excluded from analysis those subjects who reported never having seen a drunk person, 89 per cent of the remaining sample reported having seen a drunk person in the flesh. While the majority of these 'live' sightings had occurred in the streets, just under 16 per cent had occurred in the family home. Only 8.2 per cent mentioned the television as the source of their experience of drunk people and 2.7 per cent could not recall where they had seen drunk people.

The main point of interest in Figure 6.4 is the number of children witnessing drunkenness in the home. For this reason, a forward stepwise logistic regression was conducted in which 'at home' responses were compared with all other responses (see Table 6.6). Subsequent results revealed that children from Birmingham were less likely than those from Edinburgh to report witnessing drunkenness in the home. In contrast, those scoring high on verbal ability were less likely than low scorers to mention drunkenness in the home.

Discussion

Surprisingly, the rate at which subjects in the present study successfully identified the physical manifestations of drunkenness was slower

Table 6.6 'At home' sightings compared with all other sightings (predicting the likelihood of having witnessed drunkenness in the home)

Parameter (reference categories in brackets)	Log odds	95% C.I. ↓	↑
City (Edinburgh)			
City (2) Birmingham	2.2400	1.0600	3.4200
BPVS (low score)			
BPVS (2) high score	−1.346	−2.6926	6.004

than that reported by Jahoda and Cramond in their study. However, this was primarily due to the fact that in the current exercise the children, particularly the younger ones, were significantly slower to recognize the drunk woman than the drunk man, a contaminating factor which had not been present in Jahoda and Cramond's study design. Nevertheless, 79 per cent of the total sample required only the final section of the film in order to be successful on this task. Only eight children (3.4 per cent) failed to complete the task successfully.

While it had been predicted that subjects would be slower to attribute excessive drinking as the cause behind the woman's behaviour, it was also expected that subjects' responses to the questions *What do you think of this person – is he/she nice or not nice?* and *How do you think they are feeling – good or bad?* would also differ according to the sex of the drunk character in question. In accordance with this prediction however, the sex of the drunk character did affect the type of feelings subjects attributed to the drunk. The male drunk was more likely than the female drunk to elicit negative attributions.

Although the possibility exists that there were some subtle differences between the 'male' and 'female' versions of the films which may have contributed to subsequent differences in responses, the results discussed thus far suggest that the children, particularly those who were younger, were unfamiliar with the notion of drunkenness in women. Moreover, although as a whole the sample was generally condemnatory in their opinions of the drunk characters irrespective of the sex of character, they were more likely to attribute negative feelings to the drunk man. It would appear that although the majority of children strongly disapprove of drunkenness in any adult, and tend to attribute negative feelings to intoxicated people, there is a tendency to perceive intoxication in women to be less unpleasant or less negative in some way, or simply a different matter altogether. This latter suggestion would seem more plausible in view of the children's attitudes towards drinking by adult women, and their perceptions of female normative behaviour in relation to drunkenness (see Chapter 4).

With regard to reports of sightings of drunks, just under 65 per cent of the total sample claimed to have previously seen an intoxicated person. This was a lower figure than had been predicted. As this particular question was phrased *Have you ever seen anyone like that?*, it may have been the case that the children who had been shown the film of the drunk woman believed that they were being asked about drunk women specifically. However, there were no differences in responses in relation to sex of drunk person. Moreover, the fact that all but eight children had successfully identified drunkenness in the films suggests that responses to this question were not truly representative of children's familiarity with drunk people. Of those children who said that they had seen a person who was intoxicated on some occasion previous to this testing session, 82.6 per cent said they had encountered such an individual in the flesh, with by far the majority of these 'live' sightings occurring in the streets. Only 8.2 per cent of subjects mentioned the television as the source of their familiarity with drunks. Of particular interest was the fact that just under 16 per cent of children reported drunkenness in the home. That is not to say that drunkenness is necessarily more of a problem within these families because, as mentioned previously, young children have a tendency to associate drunkenness with alcohol consumption regardless of actual quantity consumed. It may simply be that these occasions in the home were more salient to subjects at the time of testing than other, less immediate, occasions.

With respect to the main between-subject differences, age of subject commonly appeared to be a significant factor in terms of the types of responses given. In comparison with other subjects, younger children were slower to recognize the drunk female, less negative in their attitudes towards and perceptions of the drunk character, and less likely to have seen a drunk person on a previous occasion. This age-related trend has been apparent in a number of the tasks in this study. For example, younger children have typically been found to be less knowledgeable about alcohol and drunks due in all probability to their age-limited abilities and opportunities for exposure to relevant information. Similarly, younger subjects have also been shown to hold less negative attitudes towards adult drinking in general, which ties in well with the theory that children of this young age have yet to fully develop an affective component in the context of their alcohol schemas (see Chapter 5).

With regard to the two socio-economic status groups, several differences were also observed. Middle-class subjects were slower to recognize the physical manifestations of drunkenness, more inclined to hold less negative opinions of drunks and were less likely to have previously seen a drunk than were working-class children. While it is unclear why this particular finding should emerge, it might be speculated that children from the former backgrounds may be more likely to see drunkenness from a different, possibly lighter perspective, than children from more socially deprived areas, and thus would not readily associate their previous experiences with the characterization of drunkenness depicted in the films. Alternatively, it may be that these subjects were giving what they perceived to be a calculated 'socially desirable' response.

Similarly, differences were observed when inter-city factors were examined. Subjects from both areas were equally adept in their ability to recognize the physical manifestations of drunkenness. Nevertheless, those from Birmingham were more likely than those from Edinburgh to express a negative opinion, and less likely to have previously seen a drunk person. In addition, children from Birmingham were the more likely to report incidents of drunkenness in the home. The number of persons found guilty of offences of drunkenness (including both cautions and convictions) in England and Wales for the year 1990, was 86,392 (@ 17 per 10,000 total population). The corresponding figure for Scotland was 2,820 or 5.5 per 10,000 total population. While these figures are by no means a definitive account of the incidence of drunkenness, nor do they relate specifically to the two cities under investigation, they do give some indication of the differences in the recorded occurrence of drunkenness offences between the two countries. However, the fact that this pattern of incidence contrasts with the pattern of subjects' responses suggests that some other factor or factors must be responsible for these city differences. The fact that Birmingham subjects were more likely to report drunkenness in their own homes might possibly be a contributory factor in terms of the more negative opinions held by these subjects.

Finally, comparisons with the findings reported by Jahoda and Cramond should be treated with caution because, as mentioned before, their study did not incorporate a female version of the film. In this regard the slower rate of recognition exhibited by the present sample has been discussed above. However, when responses to the question of how the drunk person was feeling were compared the current sample was slightly more likely than Jahoda and Cramond's sample to attribute negative feelings to the drunk person. Again, this may be due to the more negative attributions aimed at the female drunk in the present study. While it was not possible to conduct a similar comparison in relation to subjects' opinions of the drunk persons, this result suggests that in general young children's perceptions of drunkenness have changed little over the past twenty years.

THE DRINKING VIGNETTES TASK

In 1969, a report by MacAndrew and Edgerton was published, entitled *Drunken Comportment: A Social Explanation*. In what was to become an extremely influential piece of work within the field of alcohol studies, these authors argued that the disinhibiting effects of alcohol consumption upon behaviour were not the direct result of alcohol's pharmacological action, but rather that such effects could be understood in terms of culturally learned responses:

> People learn about drunkenness what their society 'knows' about drunkenness; and, accepting and acting upon the understanding thus imparted to them, they become the living confirmation of their society's teachings.
>
> (MacAndrew and Edgerton, 1969: 88)

Marlatt and Rohsenow (1980) conducted a comprehensive review of a series of studies which set out to test this theory. To enable comparisons to be made between the possible pharmacological effects and those socially learned effects of alcohol upon behaviour, these studies incorporated a 'balanced-placebo design', as follows: one group of subjects received a number of drinks which they were told contained alcohol and which did in fact contain alcohol; a second group received drinks which did not contain alcohol and which they were told did not contain alcohol; the third group of subjects were given drinks which they were told contained alcohol but which did not in fact contain any alcohol; and finally, the fourth group were presented with drinks which they were told did not contain alcohol, but which did in fact contain alcohol. The results of these investigations provided persuasive evidence to support the proposition that simply believing that alcohol has been consumed can induce in individuals behaviours characteristic of intoxication.

While the majority of experiments such as these have been targeted at individuals who are already drinkers, less is known about the development of alcohol-related expectancies among younger populations for whom alcohol consumption has yet to become established. However, the evidence to date suggests that relatively sophisticated expectancies are apparent in non-drinking adolescents, after which direct experience of alcohol serves to consolidate them (Christiansen, Goldman and Inn, 1982).

The emergence of expectancies in even younger children has been examined by Miller, Smith and Goldman (1990). Eighty-nine pre-dominantly middle-class boys and girls, aged from five to ten years and from the United States, participated in this study. At the beginning of the task children were introduced to a hand-puppet representing either a male or female adult, and they were told that before they had arrived this 'person' had drunk some whisky. Items from a modified version of the Alcohol Expectancy Questionnaire, which contains statements referring to possible effects of alcohol consumption, were then read out aloud to children. These children were then required to circle 'yes' or 'no' responses, depending on whether they believed that the person would experience these effects as a result of drinking the alcohol. The Alcohol Expectancy Questionnaire (Christiansen, Goldman and Inn, 1982) is designed to assess seven types of expectations about alcohol, including both positive and negative factors: (1) alcohol is a powerful agent which makes global positive transformations of experience; (2) alcohol can either enhance or impede social behaviour; (3) alcohol can improve cognitive and behavioural functioning; (4) alcohol has the ability to enhance sexuality; (5) alcohol leads to deteriorated cognitive and behavioural functioning; (6) alcohol increases arousal; (7) alcohol promotes relaxation. Analysis of subjects' responses revealed two major trends: first, the older children demonstrated more positive expectancies than the younger children; and second, there was a marked increase in the tendency to endorse positive expectancies within the eight- and nine-year-old children, in comparison with only minor shifts during the younger and older age groups. Male and female subjects did not differ in their expectancies, nor were there any differences between expectancies relating to the male puppet and those relating to the female puppet.

The study by Gaines *et al.* (1988) upon which the current exercise is based, was designed to examine young children's alcohol expectancies in more specific detail. A series of short vignettes was constructed in which the main character in each was involved in a situation which resulted in him/her having three alcoholic drinks. The three themes around which these stories were constructed were as follows: social anxiety, e.g. drinking to overcome nervousness or anxiety; celebration, e.g. drinking to enhance happiness; and escape, e.g. drinking to calm oneself after a shock. Following the presentation of the story, subjects were asked to explain why the character had the three drinks, how the character was feeling before having the drinks, and how the character felt after having the drinks. The highest possible score was given to respondents who mentioned both a psychological/emotional motive for drinking and a similar type of consequence, e.g. going to the boss's house for dinner would arouse feelings of anxiety and having several drinks would alter these feelings in some way. Not surprisingly, the results showed that the youngest children in this sample were less likely than the older children to give coordinated psychological/emotional motives and consequences. As a group, the girls also showed a higher level of performance than the boys on this task. Finally, the sample as a whole were less likely to interpret the social anxiety vignette than any of the other vignettes, in psychological/emotional terms.

The procedure for the task in the present study was similar to that employed by Gaines *et al.* (1988). Three stories incorporating each of the three themes described above were also retained. However, in addition to these a fourth vignette was included, the theme of which involved drinking for reasons of consolation, i.e. after having lost one's job. Specific details of these vignettes and the methodology of the task have been given in the methods section of this book (see Chapter 3).

Results

In the study by Gaines *et al.* (1988), a scoring system was developed whereby subjects received an overall score for their understanding of both the motivation for and consequences of drinking alcohol. This system was as follows: 0 – don't know/no response; 1 – general antecedent or consequence; 2 – specific biological antecedent or consequence; 3 – specific psychological antecedents or consequences; 4 – both psychological antecedents and consequences of drinking. However, in the current exercise the inter-rater reliability check using this scoring technique resulted in an extremely low agreement rate between the scorers (i.e. approximately 50 per cent). Following discussion between the two scorers it was decided to treat the motive questions and the consequence question separately using the following response categories for each, individually: 1 – psychological/ emotional; 2 – to get drunk/being drunk; 3 – general explanation unrelated to the specific context of the situation; 4 – physical or biological; 5 – don't know/no response.

Following the initial examination of the scores using this new criterion, agreement between the two raters was 84.6 per cent for the 'motives' responses and 82.9 per cent for the 'consequences' responses. The rationale behind the differing scores was then discussed by the two examiners, after which the rate of agreement reached was 87.3 per cent and 91.7 per cent respectively, the remainder consisting of more ambiguous responses on which the raters failed to agree.

Motives

Children's responses to the questions *Why do you think this person had three drinks of beer/whisky/wine?* and *How do you think they were feeling before they had these drinks?* were examined together, as both questions attempted to ascertain children's understanding of the motives for drinking. The best response was to give a psychological or emotional response to either or both of these questions. In total there were four main response categories for this task, more explicit details of which are given below:

Emotional/Psychological

Why did he/she have these drinks: 'To make her confident' (anxiety); 'To congratulate himself' (celebration); 'To console himself' (consolation); 'She got a bit of a fright' (escape); How was he/she feeling before having the drinks – 'sort of shy' (anxiety); 'very happy at winning' (celebration); 'downcast and miserable' (consolation); 'a bit shocked' (escape).

To get drunk

All responses which mentioned getting drunk as the motive behind drinking alcohol and which did not refer to emotional/psychological reasons at any point, fell into this category.

Normal

In this category all responses incorporated the belief that the drinking was not motivated by anything other than because the person wanted to, that is, there was no other particular reason behind this behaviour, e.g. 'she felt like it'.

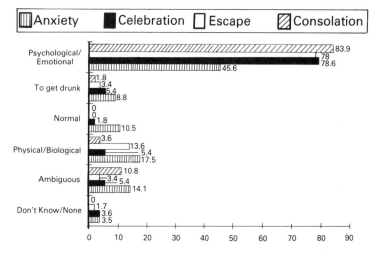

Figure 6.5 Motives for drinking

Physical/Biological

Responses in this category consisted of those in which sleepiness, thirst, etc. were put forward as motivational factors, e.g. 'he was thirsty'.

Figure 6.5 shows subjects' scores for the 'motives' questions for each of the four vignettes. For general interest, this figure also includes the proportions of subjects who gave ambiguous answers or no response at all. As can be seen from this figure, the majority of subjects gave a recognized psychological/emotional motive for the drinking for each of these situations.

Of particular interest were those subjects who had attributed a psychological or emotional motive to the drinking behaviour. For this reason, forward stepwise logistic regression was carried out, comparing subjects who had given this type of response with all other subjects. In addition, subjects' responses to the question of consequences of drinking were also included, in order to ascertain whether subjects' awareness of psychological consequences of drinking was a predictor of their awareness of psychological motives. The results of this analysis are shown in Table 6.7. It should be pointed out that due to the limitations of the statistical package used (SPSS), it was not possible to examine all interaction effects, and as a result only the main effects were included in this analysis.

Examination of the responses in relation to the particular vignette

Table 6.7 Subjects' understanding of adult motives for drinking (predicting the likelihood of giving an emotional/psychological motive)

Parameter (reference categories in brackets)	Log odds	95% C.I. ↓	↑
Vignette (anxiety)			
Vignette (2) celebration	1.9650	0.8822	3.0478
Vignette (3) escape	1.3980	0.2878	2.5082
Vignette (4) consolation	2.2650	1.1062	3.4238
Age (5–6 yrs)			
Age (2) 7–8 yrs	2.5880	1.5908	3.5852
Age (3) 9–10 yrs	3.1530	2.0382	4.2678
City (Edinburgh)			
City (2) Birmingham	1.1650	0.3532	1.9768
BPVS (low score)			
BPVS (2) high score	0.8781	0.0329	1.7233
Consequence (emotion)			
Consequence (2) other	−2.0710	−3.1316	−1.0104

subjects were presented with, revealed that the 'social anxiety' vignette was less likely than the other vignettes to elicit emotional/psychological motives for drinking. The youngest subjects, those from Edinburgh and those scoring low on the verbal fluency test were all less likely than their respective counterparts to give emotional motives, irrespective of the type of vignette. Neither the sex of the character in the vignette nor the type of alcoholic drink involved appeared to affect children's responses. However, children who gave an emotional consequence were also more likely to give an emotional motive for drinking.

Consequences

The scoring system for these responses was similar to that used for the motives responses. A few examples are given below.

Emotional/Psychological

How did he/she feel after having the three drinks of beer/whisky/wine – 'confident' (anxiety); '*very* happy' (celebration); 'sort of better' (consolation); 'a bit relaxed' (escape).

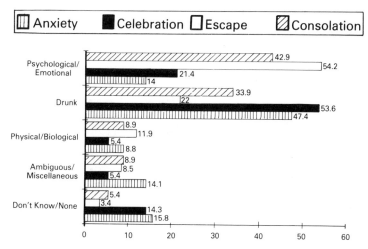

Figure 6.6 Consequences of drinking

References to intoxication

'Drunk'; 'dizzy'; 'headache and things going round', etc.

Normal

In this section, there were no responses which fell into this category.

Physical/Biological

Responses in this category referred to physical consequences other than those which were obviously associated with intoxication, e.g. 'lazy'; 'a bit better' (after being thirsty).

Figure 6.6 shows the patterns of subjects' responses in relation to the question, *How do you think the person felt after having the three drinks of beer/whisky/wine?* The most common consequence of drinking involved references to intoxication, although one-third of the sample mentioned a psychological/emotional consequence. Again, for interest, ambiguous responses and responses falling into the 'don't know/none given' category have been included in this figure.

As before, forward stepwise logistic regression was conducted in order to identify the main factors affecting subjects' performance on this question. This time, subjects' responses to the motives question were included in the analysis, in order to ascertain whether an

Table 6.8 Subjects' understanding of the consequences of drinking (predicting the likelihood of giving an emotional/psychological consequence)

Parameter (reference categories in brackets)	Log odds	95% C.I. ↓	↑
Vignette (anxiety)			
Vignette (2) celebration	0.0773	−0.9999	1.1545
Vignette (3) escape	1.7420	0.7462	2.7378
Vignette (4) consolation	1.1090	0.0916	2.1264
Type of alcohol (beer)			
Type of alcohol (2) wine	0.5640	−0.2666	1.3946
Type of alcohol (3) whisky	1.0520	0.2310	1.8730
Age (5–6 yrs)			
Age (2) 7–8 yrs	−1.2260	−2.1374	−0.3146
Age (3) 9–10 yrs	−0.6945	−1.5657	0.1767
Motives (emotion)			
Motives (2) other	−1.9130	−2.9292	−0.8968

awareness of possible psychological motives for drinking predicted an awareness of the psychological consequences of drinking. These results are shown in Table 6.8.

When the type of vignette presented was examined, it was found that the 'social anxiety' story was less likely to elicit consequences that were psychological or emotional, while the 'escape' story was most likely to provoke this type of response. In addition, a significant effect emerged in terms of the type of alcohol which the character in the vignette was drinking. Subjects were more likely to attribute psychological/emotional consequences to the drinker when the alcoholic drink was whisky in comparison to wine and then beer. As before, the sex of the character in the vignettes had no influence on the type of consequences which subjects predicted. The only between-subject factor which affected responses was age of subject. Surprisingly, it was the youngest children who were more likely to give an emotional consequence. However, this might be explained in part by the fact that the older children were more likely to give an emotional motive for drinking, and that in general those who gave such a response were also more likely then to give an emotional consequence.

Finally, the scores for the 'motives' question and the 'consequences' question were combined. The proportions of coordinated replies according to the type of vignette are shown in Figure 6.7.

Only 68 subjects (29.8 per cent) gave coordinated psychological responses. Forward stepwise logistic regression revealed no between-

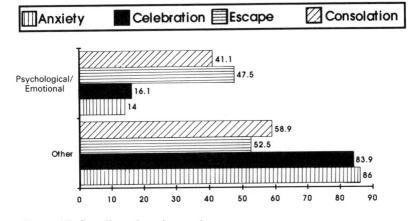

Figure 6.7 Coordinated motives and consequences

Table 6.9 Coordinated psychological responses (predicting the likelihood of giving coordinated emotional/psychological responses)

Parameter (reference categories in brackets)	Log odds	95% C.I. ↓	↑
Vignette (anxiety)			
Vignette (2) celebration	0.1553	−0.9143	1.2249
Vignette (3) escape	1.7860	0.8382	2.7338
Vignette (4) consolation	1.5470	0.5858	2.5082
Type of alcohol (beer)			
Type of alcohol (2) wine	0.9130	0.0902	1.7358
Type of alcohol (3) whisky	1.3860	0.5716	2.2004

subject differences among those who fell into this category. However, both the 'social anxiety' and the 'celebration' vignettes were less likely to elicit coordinated psychological responses, while the 'escape' vignette was most likely to provoke these types of response. In addition, when the type of drink in question was 'beer', subjects were less likely to to give coordinated psychological responses (see Table 6.9).

Discussion

This final task in the test battery was perhaps the hardest one for subjects, for two reasons. First, this was the only main activity, in contrast to the informal questioning following several of the tasks, which was dependent upon a certain level of verbal ability on the part of subjects, and which consisted of a set of unprompted, open-ended questions. Second, it attempted to measure a more subtle understanding of alcohol, in comparison to the previous tasks which assessed children's more general knowledge of this topic. Even so, very few subjects were unable to give any response following presentation of the vignettes.

With regard to children's perceptions of the motives for drinking alcohol, the majority of responses were of a psychological nature. Even so, several between-subject differences emerged. Not surprisingly, younger children and those with lower scores on the British Picture Vocabulary Scale were less likely than their counterparts to attribute psychological explanations to the subsequent drinking behaviour. These trends have been noted in several of the other tasks in this study and appear to be indicative of age-related limitations in both opportunities for social learning and cognitive ability to assimilate such information. The finding that Edinburgh subjects were less likely to give psychological explanations is more difficult to account for. The results from several of the previous tasks had indicated that children from Birmingham are somewhat less knowledgeable about certain aspects relating to alcohol, although the alcohol consumption rate per head of population in the West Midlands is somewhat higher than that for Scotland. It may be that in Scotland, drinking for motives other than emotional/psychological ones are simply more predominant, or at least more salient to young children.

When children's responses to the consequences question were examined, only one-third of the sample mentioned psychological consequences, the majority of which related to the 'escape' vignette. However, the greater proportion of responses overall referred to the intoxicating effects of alcohol, with the 'anxiety' vignette most likely to elicit this type of response. Not one subject believed that the drinker would feel 'normal' after having three alcoholic drinks. In addition, when the specific drink portrayed in the story was beer, this type of drink was less likely than whisky or wine to elicit psychological responses from the subjects.

In contrast to the motives questions, the only difference in responses according to the between-subject groups was in terms of age of subject. Surprisingly, it was the youngest children who were more likely to mention an emotional consequence. However, this was probably due to the fact that when subjects' responses to the question of motives was entered in the analysis – the majority of whom giving psychological motives being the older children – this in itself may have influenced the proceeding results.

Examination of the combined responses for both the motives and consequences questions revealed that only 29.8 per cent of the sample had given coordinated psychological responses. Interestingly, the 'social anxiety' vignette proved to be the most difficult to understand in terms of psychological/emotional motivations and consequences when considered separately and in combination. A similar finding was reported by Gaines and his colleagues (1988). It has previously been shown that the role of alcohol in the facilitation of social interaction is one that is often highlighted by many twelve-year-old children (Brown, Goldman and Inn, 1980; Christiansen, Goldman and Inn, 1982). However, it may be that for young children for whom similar concerns are yet to become important, it is less obvious to them as passive observers that an activity commonly associated with parties, gatherings, etc. should be driven by more subtle motivations. Of equal interest were responses to the 'celebration' vignette. It would appear that regardless of whether or not children attribute psychological motives for having several drinks in relation to celebrating, getting drunk is commonly perceived as an end in itself, whereas drinking for reasons of escape and, to a lesser extent, for reasons of consolation, are more readily understood in terms of alcohol's 'perceived' ability to affect emotions.

When the motives and consequences were combined, the between-subject differences which had emerged for the motive responses were no longer apparent. While this may in part be due to the fact that the majority of children from all subject subgroups referred to the intoxicating effects of alcohol when discussing the consequences of consumption, it may also partly be the result of misinterpretation of responses. It has already been pointed out that although young children do not readily reflect on the inner state of other individuals, this does not necessarily imply that they are unable to do so. Similarly, the assumption that adults interpret verbal messages from children in the way children intend them to be interpreted and vice versa can often be erroneous, especially when such open statements may contain certain ambiguous colloquialisms. Thus, in spite of the high inter-rater reliability in the scoring of responses, these results should be treated with caution.

Finally, it is worth noting that the sex of the person in the vignette exerted no discernible influence on children's responses. This is surprising in view of the evidence from the previous tasks which shows subjects' to differentiate consistently between male and female drinkers. Specifically in terms of the 'Drunkenness' task, subjects were slower to attribute intoxication as the cause behind the observed behaviour when the character in the film was female. However, Gaines *et al.* (1988) also reported no significant differences in subjects' scores between the male and female versions of the vignettes. On the other hand, the type of drink portrayed in the story did have an effect on responses. Beer was less likely than wine or whisky to be associated with coordinated psychological responses, possibly suggesting that while beer drinking is typically considered a more commonplace activity, wine and spirits or the so-called 'stronger drinks' are more readily associated with drinking to solve psychological or emotional problems.

In conclusion, it would appear that for many children, regardless of sex, social class, verbal intelligence, and so on, intoxication is the most salient consequence of consuming this amount of alcohol. It would be interesting to know whether the same pattern would have emerged were the number of alcoholic drinks to have been reduced to one or two, although there is evidence to suggest that children rarely take into account the amount of alcohol involved when considering the effects of alcohol consumption upon drinkers (Casswell *et al.*, 1988).

7 Informal survey findings

VERBAL RESPONSES: EXPERIENCE OF ALCOHOL

At specific stages during the main experimental tasks, subjects were asked a number of direct questions about their personal experience of alcohol. Both the 'Recognition of Smells' task and the 'Concept' task provided ideal opportunities for questioning children about their previous contact with alcohol, without raising their suspicion as to the true aims of the study.

Results

Recognition of Smells task

During the 'Recognition of Smells' task, subjects were asked whether they could identify, on the basis of smell, a variety of substances including two alcoholic beverages – beer and whisky. If they labelled any of the odours as alcoholic beverages, correctly or otherwise, the opportunity was taken to ask children if they had ever tasted the kinds of drinks they had mentioned and if so whether they liked or disliked them. Although thirteen children failed to identify correctly either of the alcoholic odours, eight of them did incorrectly guess that one or more of the non-alcoholic odours were alcoholic. Thus these additional questions could be asked to all but five children in the sample. Moreover, during the identification part of the task, children often mentioned alcoholic drinks other than beer or whisky. For example, on a number of occasions children mentioned drinks such as wine, sherry, vodka, etc., although in fact none of these were present. As a result, information relating to subjects' previous contact with a variety of alcoholic drinks was collected. Their responses to the question *Have you tasted (this kind of drink) before?* are shown in Figure 7.1. It is clear from this figure that the

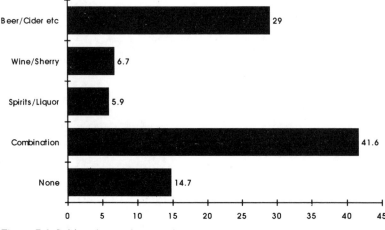

Figure 7.1 Subjects' experiences of alcoholic drinks (1)

Table 7.1 Children's experience of alcohol (1) (predicting the likelihood of having tasted one or more alcoholic drinks)

Parameter (reference categories in brackets)	Log odds	95% C.I. ↓	↑
Sex (male)			
Sex (2) female	−1.5890	−2.7900	−0.3880
Religion (Catholic)			
Religion (2) non-den.	−0.6666	−1.9586	0.6254
Ses. (m-c)			
Ses. (2) w-c	−0.9730	−1.7716	−0.1744
*Sex * Religion*			
Ses (2) * Religion (2)	1.7460	0.1050	3.3870

majority of children (*n* = 198; 85.3 per cent) claimed to have tasted alcohol, with those drinks most commonly tasted being beer, lager or cider. Forward stepwise logistic regression was performed in order to compare all subjects claiming to have tasted alcohol with those claiming not to have done so. These results can be seen in Table 7.1.

As a result of this analysis, one main significant effect emerged. That is, working-class children were less likely than middle-class subjects to have tasted one or more alcoholic drinks. In relation to the sex–religion interaction, Catholic girls were less likely than

Table 7.2 Children's likes and dislikes

	Tasted	%	Like	%	Dislike	%
Beer, lager, cider	165	54.8	78	47.3	87	52.7
Wine, sherry	49	16.3	24	49.0	25	51.0
Spirits, liquor	87	28.9	24	27.6	63	72.4
	301	100	126	41.9	175	58.1

Catholic boys to have tasted alcohol, while the sex differences for non-denominational children were not so clear-cut.

Referring further to Figure 7.1, it can be seen that a substantial proportion of subjects mentioned having tasted more than one type of alcoholic drink. For this reason, the 'combination of drinks' category was broken down in order to examine the number of subjects who mentioned having tasted each specific type of drink (see Table 7.2). Whenever subjects claimed to have tasted one or more alcoholic drinks, they were also asked which of the drinks they liked and which they disliked. The number of occasions on which subjects reported that they liked or disliked these drinks are also shown in Table 7.2.

It should be noted that when the 'combined' category of drinks was broken down, the number of children who claimed to have tasted spirits/liquor in relation to having tasted the other types of drinks was greater than had been previously indicated in Figure 7.1, although 'beers' remained the category of drinks most frequently tasted. However, it should be borne in mind that subjects were not presented with wine during this task, so the total number of subjects claiming to have tasted this type of alcoholic drink may be under-representative of their true experience of this particular type of beverage. On the whole, alcoholic drinks were more likely to be disliked than liked. This was mainly due to subjects' greater dislike of spirits/liquor ($X^2 = 10.263$; 2df; $p < 0.01$) than of beers or wines, for which responses were more or less evenly distributed between the 'like' and 'dislike' options.

The Concept task

During the 'Concept' task, a second opportunity arose to ask subjects about their previous contact with alcohol. After the main experimental section of the task had been completed and while the various bottles of alcoholic beverages were still on display, children were asked to indicate which of these kinds of (alcoholic) drinks they had

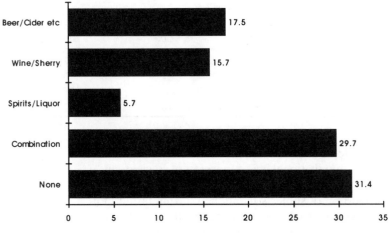

Figure 7.2 Subjects' experiences of alcoholic drinks (2)

ever tasted before. Subjects who had previously failed to demonstrate an understanding of the concept of alcohol were not excluded from this questionning, as failure to do so did not necessarily imply a general lack of awareness of alcoholic drinks. However, bearing in mind that this task took place during the second session, at which time nine subjects were unavailable for testing, the responses of the remaining 229 subjects are given in Figure 7.2.

Interestingly, on this occasion a greater proportion of the sample now claimed not to have tasted alcohol, with just over 31 per cent of the sample, saying that they had never tasted these kinds of drinks (in contrast to 15 per cent following the 'Recognition of Smells' task). However, this particular result should be treated with caution. It may be that subjects were responding to this question in terms of the specific bottles of alcoholic beverages with which they were presented, and not in relation to the type of alcoholic drink these bottles generally represented. Again, forward stepwise logistic regression was performed on these data as shown in Table 7.3.

The pattern of subjects' experience with alcohol which now emerged was quite different from that which had appeared during the previous task. Edinburgh children were more likely than the Birmingham subjects to have tasted alcohol, particularly in relation to the youngest and oldest age groups. In addition, among the middle-class subjects, those with high verbal ability were more likely than those with low ability to say they had tasted alcohol, whereas to

Table 7.3 Children's experience of alcohol (2) (predicting the likelihood of having tasted alcohol)

Parameter (reference categories in brackets)	Log odds	95% C.I. ↓	↑
City (Edinburgh)			
City (2) Birmingham	−1.0660	−2.2300	0.0980
Age (5–6 yrs)			
Age (2) 7–8 yrs	−1.4560	−2.6346	−0.2774
Age (3) 9–10 yrs	0.5834	−0.9630	2.1298
Ses. (m-c)			
Ses. (2) w-c	0.9789	0.1679	1.7899
BPVS (low score)			
BPVS (2) high score	1.1030	0.2170	1.9890
*City * age*			
City (2) * age (2)	1.4660	−0.0480	2.9800
City (2) * age (3)	−1.5250	−3.3336	0.2836
*Ses. * BPVS*			
Ses. (2) * BPVS (2)	−1.9970	−3.4230	−0.5710

Table 7.4 Children's likes and dislikes of alcoholic drinks

	Tasted	%	Like	%	Dislike	%	DK	%
Beer, lager, cider	96	38.7	70	72.9	25	26.0	1	1.0
Wine, sherry	85	34.3	62	72.9	22	25.9	1	1.1
Spirits, liquor	67	27.0	39	58.2	27	40.3	1	1.5
	248	100	171	69.0	74	29.8	3	1.2

a lesser extent among working-class children those with high ability were now less likely to have done so.

Nevertheless, the pattern of responses of those who did claim to have tasted these drinks during both tasks was similar. As before, the majority of children who said that they had tasted alcoholic drinks claimed to have tasted a variety of them, so, as before, the type of drink categories were broken down according to the number of occasions on which the drinks were mentioned. This is shown in Table 7.4, together with details of the 'like/dislike' responses.

Again, the types of drink most commonly tasted either separately or in conjunction with other alcoholic drinks were beers. However, this time, when 'wine' had actually been present during the task, a greater proportion of subjects now said that they had tasted wine and

Table 7.5 Provider of taste

	Age							
	5–6 yrs		*7–8 yrs*		*9–10 yrs*		*5–10 yrs*	
	N	%	N	%	N	%	N	%
Father only	28	50.9	25	50.0	16	30.8	69	43.9
Mother only	14	25.5	8	16.0	12	23.1	34	21.7
Both parents	7	12.7	7	14.0	13	25.0	27	17.2
Relative/friend	5	9.1	10	20.0	8	15.4	23	14.6
Self/don't know	1	1.8	0	00.0	3	5.8	4	2.5
	55	100	50	100	52	100	157	100

a smaller proportion said that they had tasted spirits or liquor than was the case following the 'Recognition of Smells' task. Also, on this occasion when not confronted with the odour of alcohol, subjects were more likely to claim to like all three types of alcoholic drink (excluding the single subject who claimed not to know), although as before, spirits/liquor elicited significantly fewer positive responses than either beers or wines ($X^2 = 11.657$; 2df; $p < 0.005$).

In addition to these questions during the 'Concept' task, subjects were examined further about their experiences of alcohol. Their responses to the question *Who gave you this/these taste(s)?* are shown in Table 7.5, excluding the seventy-two subjects who said they had not tasted alcohol.

One or both parents were commonly reported to be the initiator of children's experience of alcohol (82.8 per cent), and in particular the father was mentioned most often as the provider of the taste, either separately or in conjunction with the mother. Only one child aged five years could not remember who had provided the drink, and one eight-year-old child claimed to have been given a taste by his twelve-year-old brother. A further three children said that they had helped themselves to the alcohol.

Finally in this section, children were asked the location of this taste of alcohol. These responses are shown in Table 7.6.

Of the 113 children who said that they had tasted alcohol while at home, seven mentioned that this had also occurred while at a bar or restaurant, and one while at her aunt's house. Two children also gave a combination of responses which did not include drinking at home – one girl claimed to have drunk alcohol in a bar and in the grounds of her school, while another boy mentioned drinking at a bar and at a

Table 7.6 Location of taste of alcohol

	Age							
	5–6 yrs		7–8 yrs		9–10 yrs		5–10 yrs	
	N	%	N	%	N	%	N	%
At home	38	69.1	40	80.0	35	67.3	113	72.0
Relative/friend's home	4	7.3	5	10.0	8	15.4	17	10.8
Bar, restaurant etc.	9	16.4	4	8.0	6	11.5	19	12.1
Other*	2	3.6	0	0.0	1	1.9	3	1.9
Don't know	2	3.6	1	2.0	2	3.8	5	3.2
	55	100	50	100	52	100	157	100

* Usually an outside location, e.g. a picnic, on holiday, or during a special occasion where the location was not specified by the subject.

Table 7.7 Location of subjects' taste of alcohol (predicting the likelihood of having tasted alcohol in the home)

Parameter (reference categories in brackets)	Log odds	95% C.I. ↓	↑
City (Edinburgh) City (2) Birmingham	−1.1340	−1.8842	−0.3838
Religion (Catholic) Religion (2) non-den.	0.7453	−1.9003	1.4925

party. When subjects who mentioned tasting alcohol at home were compared with all other subjects, the following significant trends appeared (see Table 7.7). Children from Birmingham were less likely than those from Edinburgh to have tasted alcohol in the home. On the other hand, children attending non-denominational schools were more likely than those attending Catholic schools to have done so.

Discussion

As mentioned in the preceding section, the reliability of the responses to the question of experience with alcohol during the 'Concept' task should be treated with caution. A number of children (11.4 per cent) had failed to demonstrate an understanding of the concept of alcohol during the main part of the task, or had given indirect references to alcoholic drinks (21 per cent). In contrast, only five children failed to refer to alcohol during the 'Recognition of Smells' task. As explained previously, failure to demonstrate an understanding of the concept of alcohol would not necessarily imply an associated lack of awareness of alcoholic drinks in general, so these subjects were not then excluded from these additional questions. However, it may be that as a result some of these children experienced some difficulty with this line of questioning. In addition, it might be speculated that the latter task provided a more accurate reflection of direct contact simply because, while alcoholic beverages can be packaged in a variety of colours and shapes of containers, the essential odour remains constant and more distinctive. For these reasons the following discussion on subjects' experience of alcohol will be biased toward the results from the 'Recognition of Smells' task, where applicable.

The vast majority of subjects in the study (85 per cent) claimed to have tasted one or more types of alcoholic beverage, following the 'Recognition of Smells' task. This is substantially greater than the proportion documented by Jahoda and Cramond, in whose study 40 per cent of subjects claimed not to have tasted alcohol following the 'Concept' task. This was in spite of the fact that half of Jahoda and Cramond's sample had been tested following Christmas – a period during which one would expect children to be more likely to have tasted alcohol. (Even when results from the two studies were compared on the basis of the 'Concept' task the present study yielded a lower proportion of non-tasters – 31.4 per cent). On the other hand, a higher proportion of 'tasters' to that found in the present exercise, was reported by Casswell *et al.* (1983). Of Casswell's study group, 93 per cent of young New Zealand children claimed to have tasted alcohol – a figure which was confirmed by reports from the mothers of these same subjects. However, it should be noted that in Casswell's study the sample was slightly over-representative of socio-economically advantaged children, compared to the social structure of New Zealand as a whole, and in the present study, subjects from working-class areas were more likely to be among those who said that they had not tasted alcohol.

As expected on the basis of evidence from surveys of adolescents (see Chapter 2 for a review), and in accordance with Jahoda and Cramond's findings, when a sex difference occurred in the present study the boys were more likely than the girls to have tasted alcohol. In addition, working-class subjects were less likely than middle-class children to have tasted alcohol. The latter trend may be a function of the difference between parental practice, as manual workers are more likely than non-manual workers or professionals to be light drinkers or abstainers. However, these gender- and social class-related differences were found only following the 'Recognition of Smells' task. Following the 'Concept' task, the only between-subject difference to emerge between tasters and non-tasters was in terms of the two cities. It is not clear why this finding should have emerged. The fact that the population of Birmingham consists of a considerable proportion of people from Asian backgrounds who for reasons of religious affiliation and culture may be more likely to abstain from taking alcohol, may in some way account for these city differences. However, this trend may also in part be related to the finding that children from Birmingham were also less able than those from Edinburgh to group the bottles according to the alcohol/non-alcohol division during the earlier part of this task. This latter suggestion may also help to explain why the gender and class differences did not recur during the 'Concept' task, as both boys and girls, and middle-class and working-class subjects were all equally adept at the bottle-sorting task. Thus, there is added support in favour of the 'Recognition of Smells' task, as providing more accurate estimates of previous experience with alcohol.

The beverages most frequently associated with these early experiences of alcohol, accounting for just under 50 per cent of all drinks mentioned either exclusively or in conjunction with other types of beverage, were beers, lagers and ciders. This is in accordance with Jahoda and Cramond's report in which 55 per cent of subjects in their study group had tasted these types of drinks only. It is worth noting however that many young children appear to use the term 'beer' to denote various alcoholic beverages (Noll and Zucker, 1990; Fossey, 1993), and thus this figure may be over-representative of the sample's real experience of beer *per se*. Moreover in Jahoda and Cramond's study, no mention was made of combinations of drinks, making it difficult to compare results accurately or alternatively suggesting that today children are more likely to experience a wider range of such drinks. In terms of what children thought about alcoholic drinks overall, the majority of responses for all drinks fell into the 'dislike' category when degree of liking was examined following presentation of the odours. However, during the 'Concept' task, the majority of subjects said that they liked these drinks. It is likely that in the former task, the tendency for subjects to dislike the alcoholic drinks, especially spirits/liquor, is associated with the potent and off-putting odour of these drinks.

The initiator of subjects' experiences of alcohol was commonly reported to be one or both parents. On the occasions when only one parent was mentioned, it was the father who was mentioned most often. This is not surprising when one considers that married mothers constitute one of the lowest consumption rate groups (Foster, Wilmot and Dobbs, 1990). Nevertheless, the overall increase in the number of British women who do drink alcohol (Foster, Wilmot and Dobbs, 1990) may account for the fact that a relatively higher proportion of children in the present study did name their mother as the provider, either in combination with their father or separately.

As expected from looking at the provider of the taste, most children said that their experience of alcohol had occurred in their home, another trend that appears to have remained stable since Jahoda and Cramond's report. While the finding that children from Edinburgh were more likely than those from Birmingham to drink within the home might again possibly be due to differing cultural practices of the ethnic minority children in Birmingham, the reason behind the differences associated with religious affiliation is less readily discernible. One possible explanation may have been the common practice of the Roman Catholic church to present 'wine' during communion. However, this location was not mentioned by any of the subjects in connection with their alcohol experiences. Finally, although the tendency to drink outside of the home might initially give cause for concern, only two subjects gave a combination of responses which did not include drinking at home, and of these, only one gave a reply that suggested on one occasion her drinking had probably not occurred under the supervision of a responsible adult.

REPORTED STATEMENTS AND OBSERVATIONS

At various opportune points during the main experimental tasks each child was also asked a number of additional, semi-formal questions. These particular questions were included in order to assess subjects' general knowledge of alcohol and drunkenness, as well as to gauge subjects' future orientations regarding their personal use of alcohol.

Results

Children's knowledge of alcohol

As part of the 'Concept' task, subjects were presented with an array of bottles of various alcoholic drinks. After completing the main task,

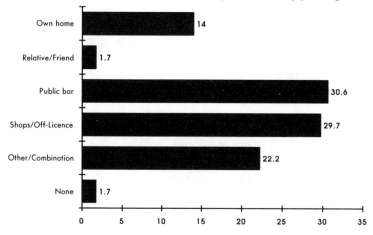

Figure 7.3 Places where bottles of alcohol sighted

children were then asked a series of additional questions. The first of these was: *Where have you seen these bottles (of alcoholic beverages) before?* Their responses are shown in Figure 7.3. The single most popular response was to mention a public bar or club. This was followed closely by 'shops', including both general stores and off-licences, with subjects' own homes being the third most common single location. However, not surprisingly a proportion of children also mentioned a combination of places where they had previously sighted bottles of this kind, their own home commonly being one of these.

When subjects were asked *Who drinks these types of drinks?*, the majority of children (51.3 per cent) made specific reference to their parents and other relatives, although one quarter of the sample widened their answers to incorporate the idea that alcoholic drinks are used by adults in general. Five children made reference to the observation that the types of people who use these drinks were typically 'drunks' or 'winos'. The remainder gave either a combination of responses or gave none at all. On further examination of subjects' responses to this question, it became apparent that many children differentiated between male and female drinkers. For this reason, Figure 7.4 illustrates subjects' responses in terms of whether they made specific mention of the sex of drinkers. As illustrated by this figure, men were considerably more likely than women to be associated with the consumption of alcohol.

During the 'Concept' task subjects were also asked *What have you*

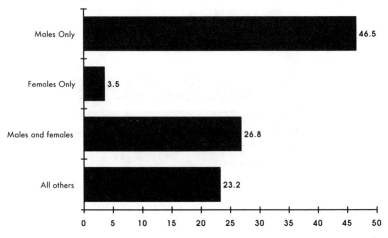

Figure 7.4 Subjects' beliefs about who drinks alcohol

been told or what have you heard about these kinds of (alcoholic) drinks? Some examples of their responses are given below, together with the total number of subjects who gave this type of response and details of the respondents who made these particular statements:

> *Positive* (n = 1): They taste good (girl aged eight).
>
> *Factual* (n = 85): They get you drunk easily, especially strong ones (girl aged ten); You can buy them from a pub (girl aged six).
>
> *Negative (a) Instructions not to drink* (n = 8): Not to drink them, not to taste them, and not to open the bottle (girl aged six); Not to have those kinds of drinks (girl aged 6); Don't drink beer (boy aged six).
>
> *Negative (b) For adults only* (n = 5): Children don't drink them, it's bad for children (girl aged eight); Only grown-ups can drink them (girl aged eight); They're not right for kids (boy aged ten).
>
> *Negative (c) Physical Harm* (n = 39): They're not good for you – you could die (boy aged ten); They're not very healthy for you (girl aged ten); When you wake up they give you a sore head (girl aged ten).
>
> *Negative (d) Miscellaneous* (n = 9): Beer's not nice (boy aged six); It's horrible (girl aged eight).

Although this question was asked in a semi-formal way, it was possible to categorize all responses into three distinct groups, as shown in Table 7.8. As can be seen from this table, the most popular response was to give a factual statement, although a substantial proportion of subjects said that they knew nothing at all about

Table 7.8 Children's knowledge of alcohol

	Age							
	5–6 yrs		7–8 yrs		9–10 yrs		5–10 yrs	
	N	%	N	%	N	%	N	%
Positive/factual	22	29.3	30	38.5	34	44.7	86	37.5
Negative	14	18.7	25	32.0	32	42.1	71	31.1
Nothing	39	52.0	23	29.5	10	13.2	72	31.4
	75	100	78	100	76	100	229	100

alcohol. Within the positive/factual category, only one subject said something positive about alcohol. In order to ascertain whether subjects differed in terms of their responses to this question, a stepwise loglinear regression was carried out. This revealed several interesting trends. First, the youngest subjects were significantly more likely than the older subjects to know nothing and less likely to know something negative, whereas the oldest subjects were more likely to know something factual. Second, in relation to verbal fluency, those who demonstrated low ability were more likely both in terms of the other subjects and the other types of response to know nothing. In contrast, those scoring high on verbal ability were more likely to give a factual response. Finally, in comparison with children from Birmingham, who were more likely to state that they knew nothing about alcohol, children from Edinburgh were more likely to say something factual. When this was further broken down by age of subject, it was found that the oldest Birmingham subjects were considerably more likely to know something negative or factual than were their counterparts from Edinburgh. The table resulting from this analysis can be seen in the Appendix 3.

Having established the type of alcohol information that subjects possessed, the source of this information was then examined. Excluding the seventy-two subjects (31.4 per cent) who had previously stated that they knew nothing, the responses of the remaining subjects are shown in Figure 7.5.

The major source of information for most subjects was either one or both of their parents. The next most popular response was that they had gained information about alcohol from the mass media. It should be pointed out that six of the children who mentioned the media also mentioned their parents. However, these were categorized under the 'media' category in Figure 7.5 simply to give a more

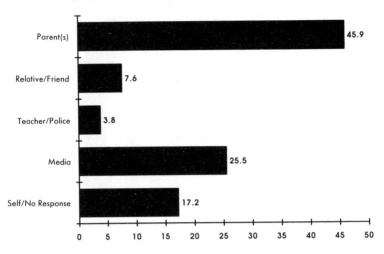

Figure 7.5 Source of information about alcohol

Table 7.9 Source of subjects' knowledge of alcohol (predicting the likelihood of having learned about alcohol from the media)

Parameter (reference categories in brackets)	Log odds	95% C.I. ↓	↑
Age (5–6 yrs)			
Age (2) 7–8 yrs	2.6600	0.5400	4.7800
Age (3) 9–10 yrs	2.881	0.7810	4.9810
City (Edinburgh)			
City (2) Birmingham	1.1020	0.2866	1.9174

realistic picture of the proportion of children who mentioned this particular source. Forward stepwise logistic regression was conducted in order to compare all subjects who gave the 'media' response (including those six who also mentioned their parents) with all other subjects. The results of this analysis are shown in Table 7.9.

Overall, the youngest children were significantly less likely than the older ones to say that the mass media were the source of their information. In addition, children from Birmingham were more likely to mention this particular source than were those from Edinburgh. There was no association between the source of children's knowledge of alcohol and the type of information they gave, although it is worth noting that children from Birmingham were both more likely to mention knowing something negative about alcohol and more likely to mention the media as being the source of this information.

Children's knowledge of drunks

A similar set of questions relating to drunk people was asked of subjects during the 'Films' task. Once subjects had established that the character in the film was acting in a drunken manner, they were then asked what they had been told or what if anything they had heard about intoxicated people. Some examples of their statements are given below:

> *Factual (n = 44)*: They just drink because they're sad (girl aged ten); They must be upset or under pressure (girl aged ten); They're alcoholics (girl aged ten); They fall over (boy aged six).
>
> *Negative (a) Instructions not to drink (n = 8)*: (You've) not to drink beer or you'll get drunk (girl aged six); When I'm big (I'm) not to drink so much (boy aged eight); (You) shouldn't drink because you'll get drunk like them (girl aged ten).
>
> *Negative (b) Instructions to avoid drunks (n = 41)*: Stay away from them (girl aged ten, boy aged eight); (I've) not to go by them (boy aged ten).
>
> *Negative (c) Drunks as dangerous or aggressive (n = 17)*: (You) shouldn't go near them as they could attack you (boy aged ten); Never go near them because they are dangerous (boy aged ten).
>
> *Negative (d) Miscellaneous (n = 19)*: They're bad for drinking whisky (girl aged six); They get silly (girl aged eight); If you see them go and tell mum and dad (boy aged ten).
>
> *Negative (e) Combined (n = 9)*: Subjects in this category gave a combination of the above types of negative statements about drunk people.

Again, these responses were divided into three categories, as shown in Table 7.10. As before, a considerable proportion of subjects (39.7 per cent) either gave no response or said that they had heard nothing about drunk people. Forty-one per cent mentioned something negative, and only 19 per cent gave some factual item of information. Not one child gave a positive statement about drunk people.

As with the question dealing with children's knowledge of alcohol, the responses to this question were analysed using stepwise loglinear regression (see Appendix 4). The same three subject factors which emerged as significant predictors for knowledge of alcohol, also

Table 7.10 Children's knowledge of drunks

	Age							
	5–6 yrs		7–8 yrs		9–10 yrs		5–10 yrs	
	N	%	N	%	N	%	N	%
Factual	14	18.7	17	21.8	13	17.1	44	19.2
Negative	14	18.7	28	35.9	52	68.4	94	41.0
Nothing/ no response	47	62.7	33	42.3	11	14.5	91	39.7
	75	100	78	100	76	100	229	100

emerged for knowledge of drunk people, namely, age, city and verbal fluency of subjects. Again the younger children were less likely to have heard anything at all about drunk people, whereas the older children, especially those aged nine to ten years, were more likely to know something negative. Factual knowledge also increased with age. As before, subjects recording low verbal fluency scores were less likely to know something factual and more likely to know something negative or know nothing at all than were the high BPVS scorers. And finally, while children from Birmingham were more likely to know nothing than were those from Edinburgh, those subjects who reported knowing something factual were more likely to be from Birmingham.

Excluding the ninety-one subjects who reported having heard nothing about drunk people, the sources of children's information about drunk people are shown in Figure 7.6. Again, the most common source for children of each age group was one or both parents, with very few children giving other positive responses. Interestingly, very few children cited the media on this occasion, in contrast to over a quarter of the subjects who mentioned this source in relation to information about alcohol.

Children's future orientations regarding alcohol

Finally in this section, subjects were asked whether they thought they themselves were likely to drink when they became older. Responses are shown in Table 7.11. Just over one-third of the sample said that they would not drink when they became older. While approximately two-fifths replied that they would drink in the future, a further 18 per cent either said that they would probably do so, or qualified their

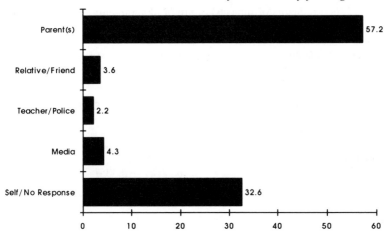

Figure 7.6 Source of information about drunks

Table 7.11 Children's future orientations regarding alcohol use

	Age							
	5–6 yrs		7–8 yrs		9–10 yrs		5–10 yrs	
	N	%	N	%	N	%	N	%
Definitely no	22	29.3	26	33.3	31	40.8	79	34.5
Possibly yes/ maybe	2	2.7	10	12.8	15	19.7	27	11.8
On special occasions	2	2.7	5	6.4	7	9.2	14	6.1
Definitely yes	47	62.7	29	37.2	17	22.4	93	40.6
Don't know	2	2.7	8	10.3	6	7.9	16	7.0
	75	100	78	100	76	100	229	100

response by indicating that they would only drink on special occasions. Only sixteen subjects were undecided as to their future drinking habits.

For the purposes of drawing comparisons between subjects, all qualified and unqualified 'yes' responses were grouped together with the 'don't know' responses. These were then compared with all 'no' responses. In addition to the standard between-subject variables such as age, sex, and so on, subjects' knowledge of alcohol and of drunk people were also entered as variables in this analysis, in order to

Table 7.12 Predictors of subjects' future drinking intentions (predicting the likelihood of children not drinking in the future)

Parameter (reference categories in brackets)	Log odds	95% C.I. ↓	↑
Religion (Catholic)			
Religion (2) non-denominational	−1.1400	−2.2958	0.0158
BPVS (low score)			
BPVS (2) high score	−2.1370	−3.4690	−0.8050
City (Edinburgh)			
City (2) Birmingham	0.5263	−0.4857	1.5383
Sex (male)			
Sex (2) female	0.7674	−0.1482	1.6830
Ses. (middle-class)			
Ses. (2) working-class	0.9645	−0.1953	2.1243
Knowledge of alc. (negative)			
Knowledge of alcohol (2) other	−1.1870	−1.9332	−0.4408
Knowledge of drunks (negative)			
Knowledge of drunks (2) other	1.2330	0.4416	2.0244
Age (5–6 yrs)			
Age (2) 7–8 yrs	0.6242	−0.2052	1.4536
Age (3) 9–10 yrs	1.3710	0.4346	2.3074
*Religion * BPVS*			
Religion (2) * BPVS (2)	1.7050	0.2120	3.1980
*Religion * Sex*			
Religion (2) * Sex (2)	1.3710	0.0150	2.7270
*BPVS * Ses.*			
BPVS (2) * Ses. (2)	2.8690	1.2400	4.4980
*City * Ses.*			
City (2) * Ses. (2)	−1.4940	−2.8546	−0.1334

ascertain whether awareness of negative aspects of drinking alcohol might also have an effect upon children's future drinking intentions. The results are shown in Table 7.12.

Looking at the main predictors only, three significant factors emerged. As expected, knowing something factual or nothing about alcohol was less likely to elicit a negative response in terms of future drinking. However, surprisingly, subjects knowing something which was not negative about drunk people were more likely to say they would not drink in the future. With regard to the demographic variables, the oldest subjects were more likely than the younger ones to say without qualification that they would not drink in the future.

Finally, in relation to the interaction effects: those with low verbal ability were more likely than high scorers to say 'no', whatever their religious affiliation but particularly among those attending Catholic schools; female subjects were more likely than boys to say 'no', again whether they attended a Catholic or a non-denominational school, although this time this trend was greater for those attending the latter type of school; working-class subjects were more likely to say 'no', whether they were of high or low verbal ability, but more so if they were of high ability; and finally in Edinburgh, working-class subjects were more likely than middle-class children to say 'no', while in Birmingham this class difference was of a smaller magnitude and in the opposite direction.

Discussion

A relatively high proportion of subjects (31.4 per cent) claimed not to have heard or not to have been told anything about alcohol, the majority of whom belonged to the youngest age group. Of the remaining subjects, most mentioned knowing something factual, and this was typically information referring to the possible intoxicating effects of alcohol consumption. Among the negative statements given, those relating to physically harmful aspects of drinking were made most frequently. Only one child said something positive about the taste of alcoholic beverages. The source of subjects' information about alcohol was commonly reported to be one or both parents, although just over one quarter of the sample referred to media sources.

Similar patterns emerged in relation to subjects' information concerning drunks, with just under 40 per cent indicating that they could recall hearing nothing about such people. Again, the majority of these subjects were from the youngest age group. The most common type of statement from subjects who did give a response was negative, and within this category most subjects recalled instructions to avoid drunks. Not one subject mentioned something positive. Again, the most popular source of this information was one or both parents, followed this time by children's own first-hand observations. Interestingly, very few children cited the mass media as the source of this aspect of their alcohol knowledge.

The between-subjects differences in terms of age, verbal fluency and city which emerged when knowledge of alcohol was examined also occurred in relation to subjects' knowledge of drunks. On both occasions the youngest subjects and those with low verbal fluency scores were more likely than their counterparts to say that they knew either nothing or something negative about these topics. These consistent patterns strongly suggest that both age-related opportunities for exposure to and developmental differences in verbal ability to assimilate this type of information are important influences on these aspects of children's knowledge. However, the fact that similar patterns were not always evident during the main experimental tasks highlights the confounding effects of asking young children questions in an open-ended format. Similarly, children from Birmingham were more likely than those from Edinburgh to know nothing about alcohol, while in relation to drunks this pattern was reversed. This latter finding complements OPCS data which indicate that the population of the West Midlands contains a greater proportion of heavy drinkers (29 per cent) than does the population of Scotland (22 per cent) as a whole (Foster, Wilmot and Dobbs, 1990). Moreover, the former trend might also be accounted for by the considerably greater proportion of ethnic minority peoples within the population of Birmingham, who as such are often likely to be affiliated to religions or cultures which advocate complete abstinence from alcohol.

Looking more closely at the kind of information children possessed, most of their statements commonly referred either to the fact that alcohol consumption leads to drunkenness or to physically harmful consequences, and that people who are drunk are generally to be avoided. In a study conducted in New Zealand by Casswell *et al.* (1983) children were asked a similar open-ended question: *What do you know about what happens to people who drink beer, whisky or wine?* In this sample too, the majority of responses concerned either the acute negative physical consequences of consumption or simply referred to the fact that alcoholic drinks induce drunkenness. Thus it may be that while the results from this and the other main tasks, e.g. the 'Drinking' vignettes task, demonstrated that many subjects in the present study, particularly older ones and those with high BPVS scores, were often aware of more subtle and more factual motives for drinking alcohol, the more negative aspects become especially salient to many children during this stage. This latter explanation certainly coincides with the overall pattern of rather negative attitudes towards adult drinking as shown in the 'Judgement of Photographs' task.

By far the most frequently cited source of children's information was one or both parents. This contrasts with evidence from a recent study by Casswell *et al.* (1988), in which children cited the mass media more often than any other source. Even so, in the present study the media were cited by just over one-quarter of the children who mentioned a source in connection with their knowledge of alcohol. These particular subjects were more likely to belong to the oldest age group, and on a number of occasions they would also mention the media in conjunction with other sources. It is worth noting that very few children referred to the provision of information about alcohol, formally or otherwise, in schools, and again, those that did tended to be older children. However, as a potential source of information about drunk people, media influence was apparent only to a very small extent. This may have important implications for the argument concerning the type of social role models for drinking depicted by the mass media, i.e. depicting excessive drinking but without the negative consequences, but is probably more likely to be due to the result of more salient first-hand sightings of drunks by subjects, overshadowing other potential learning sources.

There are a number of differences between the findings reported here and those of Jahoda and Cramond. To begin with, the number of children in the present study who did know something about alcohol (68.6 per cent) and drunks (60.3 per cent) was considerably greater than the corresponding figures in Jahoda and Cramond's sample (33 per cent and 38 per cent respectively). Furthermore in the latter study, a greater majority of responses were of a negative nature. Moreover, while parents were most likely to be the source of this knowledge in both studies, a greater number of subjects in the current study cited alternative sources, especially those connected with the media. Speculation about the nature and extent of media influence in the transmission of socio-cultural norms and values has been discussed elsewhere in this book. Nevertheless, in relation to these particular aspects of children's alcohol cognitions, the media cannot necessarily be seen as endorsing a powerful positive image of alcohol or drunkenness, in that only one subject gave positive information about alcohol, the source of which was her parents. Moreover, although the present subjects appeared to be aware of more factual aspects of consumption rather than the more negatively orientated subjects in Jahoda and Cramond's study, the type of knowledge the former possessed tended to be unrelated to their source. The only exception was with subjects from Birmingham, who, if they did know something were both more likely to know something negative about alcohol and more likely to mention the mass media as a source.

Finally in this section, children were asked about their future intentions to drink. This question was asked of subjects towards the end of the 'Concept' task but, more importantly, before the 'Drunk' films. While the majority of children in each of the three age groups stated that it was their intention to drink when they grow older, just over one-third of the study group said that they would not. Also worth noting is the fact that while children who said 'no' appeared to exhibit no element of doubt, there were varying degrees of affirmative responses. However, the fact that the vast majority of children do go on to drink alcohol during their adolescent years suggests that for many of these children such expectations are quite unrealistic, and may represent responses perceived by subjects to be 'socially desirable'. Previous research has also suggested that the older children would be more likely than the younger children to say that they did not intend to drink (Jahoda and Cramond, 1972). Indeed in the present study this was also the case, with the older subjects more likely than the younger ones to state unequivocally that they did not intend to drink. Furthermore, when sex and class differences emerged, boys and middle-class subjects were more likely to predict that they would be drinking in the future. This gender difference corresponds to the overall picture of the attitudes and perceptions of alcohol use in relation to men and women, as reflected in the main tasks of the study. In addition, both the gender and the socio-economic status differences also tie in well with evidence from adult survey data, indicating a higher incidence of alcohol consumption among men and among those adults in non-manual professions. While it is understandable that children in possession of negative information about alcohol should be less likely to predict that they would be drinkers in the future, the opposite was true when information about drunks was considered. However, the type of negative information that children had acquired about drunks was most often exhortations by parents to avoid such people. Thus it may be that young children tend not to associate themselves, as future drinkers, with these specific types of people.

In conclusion, the results from this section are interesting from a methodological point of view as well as in terms of content. A high proportion of children, especially those from the youngest age group, felt unable to give an answer to these open-ended questions relating to alcohol and drunks. In contrast, their performance on the main experimental tasks indicated that they did indeed possess some knowledge about these issues. For example, only 11.4 per cent of the sample had previously failed to demonstrate an awareness of the concept of alcohol, and an even smaller proportion (3.5 per cent) had failed to recognize the physical manifestations of drunkenness during presentation of the films. Nevertheless it could be argued that this technique of questioning is useful in that it can reveal those aspects of children's alcohol cognitions which are more salient to them, in a way that questions containing prompts of some kind are unlikely to elicit.

8 Children's perceptions of tobacco use

For the year 1991, total household expenditure on tobacco products in Britain, was just under £10,000m (Central Statistical Office, 1993). To put this into perspective, the corresponding figure for expenditure on TV and video entertainment was £7,710m and for books and newspapers etc. the total was £4,805m. However, on a more optimistic note, recent survey evidence suggests that the use of tobacco in Great Britain has shown a continual decline since 1972 (Foster, Wilmot and Dobbs, 1990). In the 1988 *General Household Survey for Great Britain*, Foster and her colleagues reported that 33 per cent of men and 30 per cent of women aged sixteen and over were current cigarette smokers, compared to the 1972 figures of 52 per cent and 41 per cent respectively. These current prevalence rates also illustrate the closing gap between the proportions of men and women who are now smokers. However, in Scotland alone, the prevalence of cigarette smoking among women is currently higher than that among men (Amos and Hillhouse, 1992).

Disappointingly, current trends in smoking habits among children are somewhat more worrying. Comprehensive information relating to smoking among British children is available from a series of surveys entitled *Smoking among Secondary School Children*. These have been conducted every two years since the first survey of this kind in 1982. The peak prevalence rates for regular smoking among school children in Britain occurred in 1984. During the following two years, the proportion of boys smoking regularly in England and Scotland had shown a decline. Although by the time of the 1990 survey, these figures remained lower than those recorded in 1984, the decrease in prevalence had now reversed. In relation to the girls, the proportion of English smokers had decreased by the time of the

1988 survey, but is now showing an upward trend. In contrast, the proportion of Scottish female smokers has shown a continuous decline. Nevertheless, the current rate of smoking among Scottish secondary-school children remains higher than that amongst pupils in England, with 19 per cent and 20 per cent of Scottish boys and girls respectively currently smoking either regularly or occasionally, compared to 15 per cent and 17 per cent of English boys and girls.

In general, it appears that although boys tend to experiment with cigarettes at a slightly earlier age than most girls, girls soon begin to catch up and may eventually overtake boys (Goddard, 1989; Currie and Todd, 1992; Loretto, 1993). For example, amongst the eleven-year-old subjects in Goddard's sample, 86 per cent of the boys and 90 per cent of the girls claimed to have never smoked a cigarette. However, by the age of fifteen years, these percentages had decreased to 36 per cent and 34 per cent respectively, with 17 per cent of boys and 22 per cent of girls now claiming to be regular smokers (i.e. smoking at least one cigarette per week). Similar findings confirming this higher prevalence of smoking among older females have been reported by a number of British studies (Foster, Wilmot and Dobbs, 1990; Goddard, 1990; MORI, 1990; Bagnall, 1991). Nevertheless, it appears that young males are still more likely than young females to be among the heavier smokers, i.e. those smoking more than ten cigarettes per day (Goddard, 1989; Goddard, 1990; Foster, Wilmot and Dobbs, 1990; Bagnall, 1991; OPCS, 1991; Loretto, 1993).

For young adolescents the key period during which initial experimentation with cigarettes occurs is typically between the ages of eleven and fourteen years. Even so, a proportion of children will have tried a cigarette at an earlier age. In Charlton's (1984) sample of schoolchildren in the north of England, 22.9 per cent of boys and 15.7 per cent of girls had already tried smoking before the age of eleven years. Although Goddard's survey of English schoolchildren indicated a decline in the proportion of 'early triers' since 1982, by 1988 17 per cent of boys and 12 per cent of girls had tried smoking by the time they were eleven years of age. Moreover, those boys and girls smoking *regularly* by the time of the 1988 survey were considerably more likely than all other subjects to have first tried smoking before the age of eleven. With regard to young Scottish children, Currie and Todd (1992) found significant regional differences among the proportions of children aged eleven years who had 'ever smoked'. These ranged from 5.9 per cent of pupils in the Borders region to 23.5 per cent for those in the Grampian region. The corresponding figure for children in the Lothian region was 16.2 per cent.

There is a consensus among studies which have examined young children's beliefs about smoking, that most young children, irrespective of whether or not they currently smoke, are very much aware of the health risks associated with tobacco use. For example, in Oei and Burton's study of seven to nine year olds in Australia (1990), 34.1 per cent of the sample claimed to have 'puffed' a cigarette. However, there was no statistical difference between the high proportion of these 'puffers' and the high proportion of those who had never tried a cigarette, who agreed that smoking was 'bad for health'. Thus, for smokers it appears that the perceived positive aspects of smoking outweigh the negative implications for health.

A second consistent finding among studies of this topic is that young children generally possess extremely negative attitudes towards the use of tobacco (Charlton, 1984; Chassin *et al.*, 1987; Goddard, 1990; Oei and Burton, 1990). In her study of 3,694 secondary-school children, Goddard reported that 82 per cent of second-year high-school children displayed negative attitudes and 18 per cent displayed neutral attitudes towards smoking, while only one subject held clearly positive attitudes towards tobacco. Of the various positive attributes that might possibly be associated with smoking the one given most credence by these subjects was 'looking grown-up'. Similarly, Charlton (1984) surveyed over 15,000 children between the ages of eight and nineteen years in the north of England. Of those older children who claimed to be regular smokers, the most common reason they put forward to explain their habit was that smoking calmed their nerves, whereas the younger smokers said that they smoked to enhance their image. In contrast, the non-smokers of the sample felt that others smoked simply to 'show off'.

While both smokers and non-smokers exhibit rather negative attitudes, there is evidence to suggest that smokers (Goddard, 1990), and female smokers in particular (Charlton and Blair, 1989), are more likely to hold slightly less negative views. Moreover, for some children, the extremely negative attitudes that they espoused when young become less disapproving over time, eventually resulting in the uptake of smoking (Chassin *et al.*, 1987; Goddard, 1990). In view of this trend it is perhaps less surprising that, by the age of fifteen years, approximately one-fifth of British schoolchildren will be regular smokers. Moreover, Goddard's data in particular suggest that the majority of these young smokers will be girls. Other variables which appear to be important predictors include having brothers, sisters and/or parents who smoke; living with a single parent; having no intention of continuing in full-time education after the age of sixteen; and finally, giving credence to the possibility of becoming a smoker in the future (Goddard, 1990).

Jahoda and Cramond's study did not incorporate any questions relating to actual use of tobacco by subjects. However, two of the tasks did present the opportunity of examining children's attitudes towards and perceptions of normative tobacco use. In brief, their results confirmed that young children were strongly disapproving of smoking. In addition, these subjects tended to attribute a significantly greater disliking of this activity to children than to adult men and women.

Although the present study was primarily concerned with young children's alcohol cognitions, two of the tasks also incorporated several items designed to elicit information relating to their ideas about tobacco use. These tasks were (1) the 'Judgement of Photographs' – designed to elicit subjects' attitudes towards adult use of tobacco, and (2) the 'Perceived Likes and Dislikes' task – designed to examine subjects' perceptions of what constitutes normative smoking behaviour in men, women and children. In this chapter, the results from these two tasks are described in detail, followed by a discussion of the findings.

Results

Children's attitudes towards adult smoking

Included in the sets of photographs presented to subjects during the 'Judgement of Photographs' task were several photographs of either men or women engaged in one of two smoking-related activities. In the case of the women, this activity was smoking a cigarette, while the men were shown either smoking a cigarette or smoking a pipe. Attitude scores for the smoking items were derived according to the same procedure as that used to derive attitude scores for the alcohol items, as outlined in Chapter 3. Thus, in the following table a score of below 40 indicates a positive attitude and a score of above 40 indicates a negative attitude towards smoking, with 70 being the maximum score possible. Table 8.1 shows the attitude scores for all subjects in relation to each smoking item. It can be seen from this table that the sample as a whole held distinctly negative attitudes towards smoking a cigarette. Attitudes towards pipe smoking were also clearly negative, but slightly less so than attitudes towards cigarette smokers. As mentioned above, only men were depicted smoking a pipe in these photographs.

Table 8.1 Attitudes towards adult smokers by age of subject

	Age							
	5–6 yrs		*7–8 yrs*		*9–10 yrs*		*5–10 yrs*	
	Mean	*SD*	*Mean*	*SD*	*Mean*	*SD*	*Mean*	*SD*
Cigarettes								
Men	50.63	12.96	56.69	10.23	58.80	11.53	55.39	12.06
Women	50.33	12.23	55.08	11.28	57.26	10.38	54.24	11.64
Both	50.45	11.32	55.65	10.25	58.08	10.14	54.74	11.00
Pipe								
Men	48.30	10.59	51.51	9.18	50.97	8.47	50.27	9.52

Table 8.2 Subjects' attitudes towards smoking a cigarette

	SS	DF	MS	F	SIG (P)
Between subjects					
Within cells	29406.34	146	201.41		
Constant	1316197.05	1	1316197.05	6534.81	0.000
Age (A)	4960.51	2	2480.26	12.31	0.000
Sex (B)	602.37	1	602.37	2.99	NS
Ses. (C)	9.96	1	9.96	< 1	NS
City (D)	284.26	1	284.26	1.41	NS
Religion (E)	31.92	1	31.92	< 1	NS
BPVS (F)	1571.24	1	1571.24	7.80	0.006
Within subjects					
Within cells	4587.12	146	31.42		
Gender (G)	115.08	1	115.08	3.66	NS
B * G	709.53	1	709.53	22.58	0.000

Separate analyses were carried out on both of these smoking items, in order to identify which, if any, factors may have influenced subjects' attitudes. Table 8.2 shows the results of a multivariate analysis for the item 'smoking a cigarette'. To minimize presentation of these results, only those interactions which were significant have been included in the tables.

As age of subject rose, attitude scores for 'smoking a cigarette' became increasingly negative, although it should be stressed that even the youngest children demonstrated quite clearly negative attitudes. In addition, subjects who recorded above average scores on

Table 8.3 Subjects' attitudes towards smoking a pipe

	SS	DF	MS	F	SIG (P)
Source of variation					
Main effects	1245.64	7	177.95	2.012	NS
Age (A)	452.45	2	226.23	2.558	NS
Sex (B)	9.55	1	9.55	< 1	NS
Ses. (C)	512.02	1	512.02	6.789	0.017
City (D)	105.53	1	105.53	1.193	NS
Religion (E)	8.99	1	8.99	< 1	NS
BPVS (F)	3.27	1	3.27	< 1	NS
2-way interactions	2048.19	1	2048.19	1.16	NS
B * C	358.46	1	358.46	4.05	0.046

the British Picture Vocabulary Scale held more negative attitudes than did low scorers, towards cigarette smoking. Whether the person smoking was male or female did not significantly affect overall attitudes. However, female subjects were more negative when the person shown smoking in the photograph was a woman.

A single anova was carried out for the item 'smoking a pipe', as only men were depicted in these photographs. The results of this analysis can be seen in Table 8.3. Attitudes scores for this activity did not differ significantly in relation to age of subject. In fact, the only significant main effect to emerge from the analysis was in terms of social class. Middle-class children, and in particular middle-class boys, were more disapproving than working-class children of smoking a pipe.

Figure 8.1 illustrates the sample's attitudes towards smoking in general with those towards alcohol. It can be seen that on the whole, the smoking activities elicited more extreme negative attitudes from the sample, with men smoking a cigarette receiving the highest score of all.

Children's perceptions of social norms relating to smoking

The pre-recorded lists of activities presented to subjects during the 'Perceived Likes and Dislikes' task also included one or other of the two smoking-related activities, i.e. either smoking a cigarette or smoking a pipe. Thus, the lists presented to approximately half of the sample contained the item 'smoking a cigarette', while the other half of the group listened to a list of activities which included 'smoking a pipe'. On no occasion did any subject receive both the smoking items.

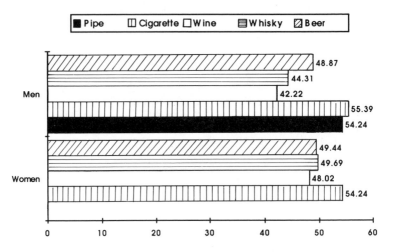

Figure 8.1 Attitudes towards tobacco and alcohol use

Table 8.4 Perceived likes/dislikes of smoking

	Age							
	5–6 yrs		7–8 yrs		9–10 yrs		5–10 yrs	
	Mean	*SD*	*Mean*	*SD*	*Mean*	*SD*	*Mean*	*SD*
Cigarettes								
Child	12.92	7.11	12.00	5.52	10.39	1.37	11.75	5.28
Woman	19.86	10.58	19.88	10.77	18.55	10.06	19.43	10.41
Man	22.64	9.96	22.75	11.21	19.74	10.19	21.71	10.49
Pipe								
Child	13.82	6.41	12.37	5.54	11.77	4.44	12.65	5.55
Woman	16.71	8.49	13.42	6.38	12.43	4.95	14.20	6.96
Man	23.55	10.89	24.34	9.53	24.86	9.01	24.25	9.78

Again, the procedure for calculating scores for the smoking items was the same as that used for the alcohol-related items in this same task. Thus, in the following tables, scores range from 10 (maximum dislike) to 40 (maximum liking), with 25 being the neutral point.

Looking at the overall scores for the group as a whole, it should be emphasized that subjects perceived all three roles (i.e. men, women

Table 8.5 Perceived likes/dislikes of smoking a cigarette

	SS	DF	MS	F	SIG (P)
Between subjects					
Within cells	4543.06	45	100.96		
Constant	92499.12	1	92499.12	916.22	0.000
Age (A)	424.19	2	212.10	2.10	NS
Sex (B)	143.28	1	143.28	1.42	NS
Ses. (C)	319.93	1	319.93	3.17	NS
City (D)	181.09	1	181.09	1.79	NS
Religion (E)	10.48	1	10.48	< 1	NS
BPVS	850.33	1	850.33	8.42	0.006
Within subjects					
Within cells	4019.44	90	44.66		
Identity of smoker					
(G)	4998.85	2	2499.42	55.96	0.000
B * G	337.15	2	168.58	3.77	0.027

and children) to dislike both smoking activities, although to varying degrees. A general pattern emerged, with the greatest perceived dislike for smoking both a cigarette and a pipe attributed to children. Less extreme dislike for both of the activities was attributed to women, although in relation to pipe smoking this occasionally reached a similar level to that attributed to children. Finally, men were perceived as disliking these activities least.

Table 8.5 shows the results of the multivariate analysis of variance for 'smoking a cigarette'. In general, children attributed greater dislike of smoking to children than they did to either men or women. In addition it was found that the female subjects attributed greater dislike of smoking to young girls than did the male subjects to young boys. Finally, subjects who had previously attained a high score on the British Picture Vocabulary Scale perceived greater general dislike of smoking a cigarette than did those with lower scores.

Looking at Table 8.6 it can be seen that perceptions relating to smoking a pipe were quite unaffected by any of the six between-subjects factors. However, liking scores did differ in terms of the type of smoker involved. As expected, children attributed less dislike of smoking a pipe to men than they did to women or children.

Finally, Figure 8.2 shows subjects' perceived likes/dislikes for both the smoking-related items and the alcohol-related activities. In comparison to drinking any of the three types of alcoholic beverage,

Table 8.6 Perceived likes/dislikes of smoking a pipe

	SS	DF	MS	F	SIG (P)
Between subjects					
Within cells	3462.50	44	78.69		
Constant	94627.08	1	94627.08	1202.48	0.000
Age (A)	193.98	2	96.99	1.23	NS
Sex (B)	43.96	1	43.96	< 1	NS
Ses. (C)	9.63	1	9.63	< 1	NS
City (D)	10.19	1	10.19	< 1	NS
Religion (E)	147.79	1	147.79	1.88	NS
BPVS (F)	18.51	1	18.51	< 1	NS
Within subjects					
Within cells	3658.33	88	41.57		
Identity of drinker (G)	8955.29	2	4477.64	107.71	0.000

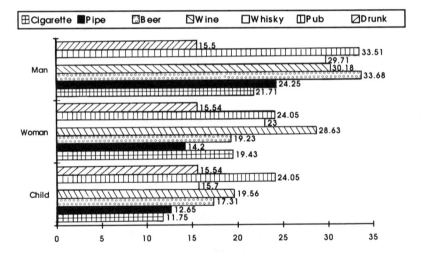

Figure 8.2 Perceived likes/dislikes of tobacco and alcohol

subjects' perceived dislike of smoking either a cigarette or a pipe was considerably greater. The only exception to this trend was subjects' more negative attributions for women drinking beer. However, 'being drunk' remained the activity most commonly perceived to be disliked by men, women and children overall.

Discussion

Overall, subjects displayed extremely disapproving attitudes towards smoking in general, although cigarette smoking elicited slightly more negative attitudes than did pipe smoking. Likewise, children's perceived dislike of such activities was also high, particularly when these were associated with young children like themselves. Again, a difference emerged in relation to the two types of smoking activity, with less dislike of pipe smoking than of cigarette smoking being attributed to men. Despite being generally more negative about tobacco use in comparison to alcohol consumption, the pattern of subjects' responses to both of these types of activity were very similar.

With regard to cigarette smoking, attitudes towards this activity were distinctly negative even among the youngest children, although they became more disapproving as age of subject increased. As with the oldest children, those subjects who displayed greater verbal fluency on the British Picture Vocabulary Scale were also more disapproving than low scorers of smoking a cigarette. These children also gave higher perceived dislike scores than did low scorers, irrespective of whether the smoker was a man, woman or child. Alternatively, there were no corresponding age differences in relation to children's like/dislike attributions. All three subject age groups attributed similar levels of dislike for smoking a cigarette, nor did attitudes differ according to the gender of the smoker.

The finding that there were no main differences between subjects' attitudes towards male and female cigarette smokers was particularly interesting. A similar finding also emerged in relation to their attitudes towards beer drinkers (see Chapter 5), in which subjects were more negative about beer drinking generally and did not distinguish between male and female drinkers. However, when the possible influence on performance of the type of person engaged in smoking a cigarette was considered in association with the gender of subject, a significant trend did emerge. First, just as girls had previously been found to be more condemnatory of female beer drinkers, in the current task it was found that girls were also particularly disapproving of female smokers. In addition, while children generally attributed a greater dislike of smoking to children than they did to adults, girls perceived greater dislike for smoking than boys when the role was that of a child of the same sex. Unfortunately, it was not possible to perform a cross-sex comparison to examine whether these children either did in fact perceive a real difference between the preferences of girls and boys, or that girls were simply more disapproving than boys in general, of tobacco use.

Also of interest was the fact that subjects' attitudes did not differ in terms of social class. Although the OPCS surveys of children do not collect data corresponding to social-class differences, data relating to adults have shown a higher prevalence of smoking among manual workers than those in non-manual professions. However, information of this kind in relation to Scottish children has been examined by Currie and Todd (1992). These authors found that of the female smokers in their sample, those whose fathers were in manual employment (17 per cent) were significantly more likely than those whose fathers were in non-manual professions (12 per cent) to be current smokers. For this reason it might reasonably have been expected that the working-class children in the present sample would be less disapproving of smoking in adults. However, this was not the case. Moreover, despite the fact that the prevalence of cigarette smoking is somewhat higher in Scotland than in Great Britain as a whole, for adults and adolescents, both males and females (Amos and Hillhouse, 1992), there were no corresponding differences in the attitudes and perceptions of smoking among the present study group.

In general, subjects' scores with regard to smoking a pipe were more or less uniform, with the exception of social class. Children from middle-class backgrounds were more disapproving than those from working-class backgrounds. Data from the 1991 OPCS survey have indicated that while cigarette smoking is lowest among adults in non-manual occupations and highest among those in manual occupations, there are no such differences in relation to pipe smoking. Indeed Goddard (1989) found that only 4 per cent of the adult men in her sample claimed to be pipe smokers. However, the finding in the present study does suggest that, at least for this study group, pipe smoking may be more predominant among the middle classes, and is therefore of greater issue to these particular children. With reference to subjects' perceptions of the social norms for pipe smoking, these results revealed no differences between subjects. However, as expected, children attributed less dislike of smoking a pipe to men than they did to women and to children.

The early development of both attitudes and norm perceptions in relation to alcohol has been discussed in greater detail in Chapter 5, and for this reason, few additional comments will be mentioned here. However, there are two points which should be highlighted. The first is that children of this age range evidently consider the use of tobacco to be less acceptable and of more serious concern than the use of alcohol. The source and content of didactic messages concerning alcohol, both on a personal level and on a policy level, are varied and often conflicting. In contrast, similar messages relating to the harmful effects of tobacco are on the whole less confused and therefore more coherent to young children. Thus, unlike the almost neutral attitude scores of the youngest children following the 'alcohol' version of the 'Judgement of Photographs' task, their scores on the 'tobacco' version of this same task indicate more clearly established attitudes. Moreover, the tendency of the sample as a whole not to differentiate between male and female smokers reinforces the idea that smoking under any circumstance, and by any person, cannot be condoned.

This leads on to the second issue, which concerns the recurring theme of sexual stereotyping, and in particular that exhibited by the girls in the sample. As mentioned above, it is difficult to be certain as to the explanation behind the female subjects' stereotypical responses in the 'Perceived Likes and Dislikes' task. Do they reflect a genuine perception of gender-based differences or are they simply due to the fact that girls perceive tobacco and alcohol use in a more negative light than do boys? The finding that girls are generally particularly disapproving of female smokers when asked to judge both male and female adult smokers suggests that the former explanation may be closer to the truth.

Finally, there is some evidence that children's ideas about smoking may have changed a little over the last twenty years. The negative attitudes of the younger children in the present study were relatively more pronounced than those of their age counterparts in Jahoda and Cramond's sample. Thus it appears that the more recent introduction of nationwide campaigns against smoking are not only achieving success in terms of an overall decline in adult smokers, but are also continually reinforcing in children from an early age negative messages concerning tobacco. This is echoed in the findings of several studies assessing the impact of smoking education on young children, in which modest positive achievements have been noted both in terms of the young children themselves (Wilcox and Gillies, 1981; Gillies and Wilcox, 1984) and in relation to their parents (Wilcox *et al.*, 1981). In contrast, the tendency for girls to be more disapproving of female smokers appears to be a persistent one. This trend was observed in both the present exercise and the study conducted by Jahoda and Cramond. It is more difficult to draw similar conclusions in terms of the perception scores as these data were treated differently by the authors. In the current study, analysis was carried out on the two smoking items separately, whereas Jahoda and Cramond combined the 'smoking a cigarette' and 'smoking a pipe' items in their analysis. Nevertheless, it appears that in comparison to the subjects in the original exercise, the children in the current study generally tended to perceive greater dislike of these smoking activities.

9 Conclusions and recommendations

THE MAIN FINDINGS

Since the publication of Jahoda and Cramond's report in 1972, additional research into the development of young children's alcohol cognitions has been noticeably scarce. The assumption that children are innocent with regard to alcohol, and would therefore constitute a somewhat irrelevant area of study, has probably been the major barrier to investigation of this topic. Opinion, both then and now, remains heavily influenced by this belief. Parents, too, commonly assume ignorance on the part of their children (Fossey and Anderson, 1993). However, the findings of the present study suggest that in Britain a substantial number of children will have tasted alcohol well before their teenage years. While this apparent divergence between opinion and practice may in part be due to a generational shift in parental conduct with regard to alcohol and young children, it is more likely to be due to imprecise recollections of parents' own early experiences with alcohol. As has been remarked upon elsewhere in this book, personal accounts of the age at which initial contact with alcohol occurred tend to increase as a function of age.

It might also be argued that young children may be over-reporting the extent of their direct experiences with alcohol. The difficulties involved in interpreting children's responses to what may be perceived to be socially sensitive questions have been discussed in Chapter 1. However, it was for this reason that the present study was primarily designed to provide objective results, placing as little reliance on direct verbal questioning as was possible. With such a young age group, it was not possible to assess directly the extent of children's personal contact with alcohol, as this would have necessitated asking subjects to taste alcoholic drinks. Instead, under these circumstances, a test involving the recognition of alcoholic odours provided the best alternative strategy. The results of the 'Recognition of Smells' task, having first accounted for shortcomings in ability to identify odours *per se*, revealed extremely high levels of familiarity with alcohol. Only thirteen children (5.5 per cent) were unable to identify either one of the two alcoholic beverage odours. This finding indicates that familiarity with alcohol is indeed a pervasive phenomenon among young children, at least within the two study areas, although this was less likely to be the case in relation to the youngest subjects. Moreover, because the methodological design of this task was such that the possible influence of age-related differences in cognitive ability was minimized, the results suggest that these small but significant age-related differences in performance were largely attributable to corresponding differences in exposure to alcohol.

Although the two alcoholic beverages involved in the odour task – beer and whisky – were identified by similar numbers of children, there was a clear trend for subjects to use the term 'beer' to denote either of these drinks. This tendency to use specific names of alcoholic beverages as a generic term incorporating all such drinks was again highlighted in the 'Concept' task. Only twenty-six children (11.4 per cent) failed to demonstrate some awareness of the conceptual difference between alcoholic drinks and other drinks. However, while the majority of the oldest children were both more likely to separate the eight bottles according to the alcohol/non-alcohol division and were more likely to apply the correct verbal label to this concept (i.e. 'alcohol'), for the sample as a whole, the most popular method of describing this difference was in terms of names of specific alcoholic drinks (i.e. 'they're all beers').

The proportion of subjects who demonstrated an awareness of the operational concept of alcohol was 88.6 per cent. Whereas nearly all of the subjects from the two older age groups were able to do so following assistance from the experimenter, a slightly, but nevertheless significantly, smaller proportion of the youngest subjects (81.4 per cent) were also successful. Performance on the preceding training trial, i.e. the 'fruit/non-fruit' task, indicated that all but eight subjects understood the idea of category concepts. Moreover, failure to understand the fruit/non-fruit groupings was not a predictor of failure to perform the alcohol/non-alcohol groupings. Thus it would appear that, while children as young as five and a half years are cognitively able to categorize objects according to an accepted set of ideas, their performance will inevitably be dependent upon their familiarity with the objects in question and the category which they constitute. The finding that the verbal explanation applied to the alcohol groupings also differed according to the age of subject provides further support of this. In addition, although the majority of all subjects were able to apply correctly the term 'fruit' to the food groupings, a considerably smaller number ($n = 61$; 30 per cent) referred to the term 'alcohol' in relation to the bottles, only one of whom belonged to the youngest age group. Thus, while the operational concept of alcohol appears to become established at around six or seven years of age, the verbal concept appears at a slightly later age, when children are approximately eight or nine years of age.

Subjects' understanding of the consequences of consuming alcohol was examined by two of the tasks in the study. The rate at which subjects recognized the physical manifestations of heavy alcohol consumption during the 'Drunkenness' films task was extremely high. In fact, children were as familiar with drunken comportment as they were with the odour of alcoholic beverages. The finding that most subjects were able to pinpoint the cause behind the behaviour they were viewing, despite the fact that additional sound cues were not present, suggests that most children are aware of the intoxicating effects of alcohol upon adult behaviour, although again it was the youngest children who were less likely to be able to do so. In contrast, children's understanding of the possible psychological motives and consequences of consumption, as measured by the 'Drinking' vignettes task, was less well developed. This is not surprising in that emotional expectations with regard to alcohol are by definition less readily observable to young and old alike and thus require more subtle understanding. It should also be re-emphasized that there was a certain amount of disagreement between the two raters in relation to the children's scores on the 'Drinking' vignettes task. This highlights the problem of interpretation between child and adult communications. It might be that in some cases the child's response was misinterpreted by the raters. For example, although some children may in fact have possessed a degree of understanding of the psychological motives and/or consequences of drinking, they may have been unable to convey this succinctly to the experimenter. There is also the possibility that children were unsure of the questions asked of them. Finally, with regard to the consequences of consumption specifically, physical intoxication may not have been the only consequence known to children, but simply the most salient one, especially considering that fact that the theme of drunkenness had been covered in the immediately preceding task. For these reasons it is difficult to make decisive statements on the basis of these results. However, it is possible to conclude tentatively that, while most children in this study group were familiar with drunken comportment by the age of five and a half, an understanding of the perceived psychological effects of consumption appears to develop at a slower rate.

The remaining tasks presented to children in this study were designed to produce indirect measures of subjects' perceptions of the norms relating to alcohol use by men, women and children, and their attitudes towards adult use of alcohol. With regard to the former, children appeared to have quite well-established ideas about what constitutes normative drinking behaviour with particular reference to adult male and female drinkers. The consumption of all three types of alcoholic beverage was perceived to be very much the preserve of adult males, although subjects did attribute a liking of wine to women. Moreover, these perceptions did not differ with respect to the age of subjects. However, this was not the case when subjects' attributions for children were considered. Although even the youngest subjects were able to distinguish between the degrees of inappropriateness of drinking alcohol by children and by adults, the older children tended to advocate this more strongly.

In contrast, children's attitudes towards adult drinkers did differ in relation to age of subject. Irrespective of both the gender of the drinker and the type of alcoholic beverage consumed, as age of subject rose children became increasingly negative towards drinkers. Together, these findings suggest that, while many young children are aware of differences in normative adult drinking, either the ability or the propensity to make moral judgements about these behaviours develops at a later stage. Examination of children's attitudes towards adult smokers strongly suggests that even the youngest children were well aware of the negative value placed by many key 'authority figures' upon tobacco consumption. Young and old subjects were extremely disapproving of all smokers, although again the older children were even more so. Thus the results suggest that while young children do have the ability to make critical judgements about certain activities, at this stage, the intensity with which these attitudes are held increases as older children become more 'socially aware' of the implications and thus are more likely to make internalized moralistic judgements.

Sexual stereotyping

Although boys and girls tended not to differ in their levels of knowledge of alcohol, their interpretations of drinking norms and their attitudes towards adult drinkers did show marked differences. In addition, whenever the tasks necessitated subjects to differentiate between men and women in association with various drinking activities the sample as a whole likewise reflected these differences in their responses.

The first task which presented subjects with the issue of gender was the 'Judgement of Photographs' task. Although the children did not differ significantly in their attitudes towards male and female beer drinkers, both the female whisky drinkers and the female wine drinkers elicited greater disapproval than did their male equivalents. This bias was also in evidence during the 'Perceived Likes and Dislikes' task. On this occasion, while men were perceived to like all but one of the alcohol-related activities, women were perceived to like only drinking wine. While it might be argued that these children were only distinguishing between males and females because they were presented with the opportunity to do so, their spontaneous responses to the informal question *Who normally drinks these kinds of (alcoholic) drinks?* (see Chapter 7) suggest that this is not the case. Finally, further objective evidence of this stereotypical effect emerged during the 'Drunkenness' task. Following the presentation of the films, it became apparent that the female drunk was likely to cause subjects difficulty in terms of attributing drunkenness to the observed behaviour; whereas those subjects who had been presented with the 'male' version of the film were markedly quicker at understanding the theme. In fact, the only task in which a sex of character effect was not apparent was following the 'Drinking' vignettes task.

Taken together, these findings suggest a reluctance on the part of young children to associate with women a variety of alcohol-related activities. Of particular interest were subjects' responses to the idea of drinking wine. This item had been introduced to the present study as an example of a less stereotypically male activity. However, while on the one hand subjects acknowledged that drinking wine was as normal an activity for women as for men, they evidently disapproved of women doing so. Nor could this trend be attributed solely to the double-standard of the boys, as it transpired that it was the girls who were the more judgemental. That is, not only were the female subjects often more likely to disapprove of both male and female drinkers and more likely to attribute greater dislike of such activities to both, but they were also more likely than boys to disapprove of, and perceive greater dislike on the part of, female drinkers in particular. This tendency was also apparent in the girls' perceptions of norms relating to young girls like themselves. Girls were more likely to attribute a general dislike of alcohol-related activities among girls than were boys in relation to other boys.

Speculation as to why this sex-stereotyping should occur has been documented in greater detail in Chapter 5. However, in brief, it appears that both the type of information children acquire and the way in which they assimilate this are factors which may be responsible. Contrary to the common belief that women are now more likely to be considered as the equals of men in relation to many issues, e.g. education and employment opportunities, most of the literature pertaining to the consumption of alcohol appears to negate this. A persistence in the stereotype that women who drink and get drunk are somehow more worthy of reproach than men has been reported by several studies of young adults (Fillmore, 1984; Snortum, Kremer and Berger, 1987; Landrine, Bardwell and Dean, 1988). Nevertheless, a more recent study by Lang, Winiarski and Curtin (1992) suggests that the situation may be changing. The perceptions of a study group of undergraduates in the United States were found not to differ in relation to male and female drinkers. However, the finding that these same students were also more likely to be positive in their perceptions of non-drinkers, in opposition to their own drinking habits, might be suggestive of an inclination to give what might be perceived to be 'politically correct' responses.

The findings of this present study are important if they imply that girls internalize some form of guilt or shame about drinking. Perhaps there still exists a perceived discrepancy between the behavioural norm for women drinkers and the view that this is somehow at odds with the traditional female role. It has also been suggested that women with alcohol problems are often deterred from seeking help, due to this stigma. Alternatively, there may be a more simple and less sinister explanation for these stereotypical responses. With regard to the younger age under consideration in this study, at this early stage children are only just beginning to develop ideas about alcohol in relation to their own gender schemas. In order for this incoming information to make sense to them and to provide a satisfactory basis of knowledge on which to expand and adapt further information as it is assimilated, these early schemas are necessarily very simplistic and thus appear highly stereotyped.

Further subject group differences

A number of trends also emerged in relation to other between-subject variables. Two of these in particular deserve some mention.

Between-city differences

There are a number of differences between England and Scotland in relation to patterns of alcohol consumption. Despite common lay opinion concerning the alleged drinking excesses of Scottish people, the proportions of drinkers and of heavy drinkers are greater in England. So too is the reported incidence of criminal convictions relating to intoxication. Perhaps for these reasons it might have been expected that children from Birmingham would have shown an overall greater awareness of alcohol. However, this was not necessarily always the case. In fact, subjects from Edinburgh were not only more likely to have tasted alcohol than were those subjects from Birmingham, but they also tended to know more about alcohol and drunkenness, the latter often by way of first-hand observations. Thus, it may be that definitions of 'drinking culture' which are based upon gross epidemiological variables are failing to capture the more subtle factors involved.

Although ethnic background was not treated as a separate factor within this study, it was apparent that, while the Scottish sample consisted of only very few children from Asian backgrounds, the Birmingham sample contained children of diverse ethnicity. While it is not possible to draw definitive conclusions on the sole basis of this difference with regard to this particular study group, it is likely that the unexpected trends in these results are due to the differing religious and cultural practices of these subjects, which commonly advocate abstinence. Thus, it might be speculated that had the religiosity division been in terms of a religion other than Roman Catholic, this factor might have emerged as a more significant predictor overall. As it was, religious affiliation, as differentiated in this study, appeared to have very little influence on children's responses.

Social-class differences

Further differences in performance also emerged in relation to the socio-economic variations between subjects. These differences were generally in the direction predicted, bearing in mind that children from the middle-class areas were also more likely to possess greater verbal/cognitive ability than were children from more working-class backgrounds. In particular, the attitudes and norm perceptions of middle-class children often mirrored those of the older subjects and those with high British Picture Vocabulary scores, suggesting that these groups of children had the greater opportunity and a more highly developed cognitive capacity to assimilate information relating to most of the aspects of alcohol covered in this study. Similarly, working-class *adults* are more likely both to abstain from drinking and indulge in tobacco smoking.

Comparisons with the findings of Jahoda and Cramond

It was hypothesized that the recent increases in both the proportion of British adult drinkers and per capita consumption of absolute alcohol might be reflected in the performance of subjects in this new exercise, compared with that of Jahoda and Cramond's study group. Moreover, the opportunities which exist for children to learn about alcohol are now highly pervasive. In Britain currently, over 90 per cent of adults consume alcohol to some extent, millions of pounds are spent by the alcohol industry on sponsorship and on the advertisement and promotion of alcoholic beverages through the mass media, and a considerable amount of time on television and films involves the depiction of drinking. Finally, the inclusion within the school curriculum of some element of alcohol education has become more widespread since the time of the original study.

On observing the significantly greater familiarity with alcohol demonstrated by the present subjects during the 'Recognition of Smells' task, it would seem reasonable to infer that this reflects the widespread increase in alcohol consumption since the early 1970s. Unfortunately, the methodological differences between the two studies make it difficult to draw decisive conclusions on this basis alone. However, if one goes on to consider the between-study differences in knowledge of both alcohol and drunkenness (Chapter 7), one finds further evidence to substantiate this claim. In both instances, a significantly greater proportion of children in the current investigation were able spontaneously to demonstrate a basic knowledge of alcohol and its intoxicating properties.

While there was little difference in the proportions of older children who showed an awareness of the concept of alcohol between the two studies, a significantly greater proportion of the youngest children in the present exercise were familiar with this operational concept. Similarly, there was an increase in the number of children who applied the term 'alcohol' to this concept among the present study group. In fact, the only apparent exception to this overall recent trend of greater familiarity with alcohol emerged following the 'Drunkenness' task. On this occasion, the current sample were noticeably slower in their ability to recognize drunken comportment. Even so, this difference can again be accounted for in terms of methodology. The slower rate of recognition was primarily due to the difficulty with which children were confronted when presented with the film of the intoxicated woman, a confounding factor which had not been present in the same task by Jahoda and Cramond.

Finally, several differences emerged in relation to children's subjective perceptions of normative drinking behaviour and attitudes towards drinkers. In the former study, subjects perceived a greater degree of liking of alcohol among men and less dislike among women and children. While these current perceptions appear more realistic in terms of recent trends in consumption, they remain vastly under-representative of adults' true drinking preferences. It has been mentioned elsewhere in this book that married mothers constitute one of the lowest consumption groups. Moreover, married fathers are also more likely to report low or very low consumption rates compared with other married or single men (Foster, Wilmot and Dobbs, 1990). It might thus be speculated that parents of young children provide differential standards of 'normative' drinking behaviour.

With regard to between-study changes in attitudes towards drinkers, the only difference to emerge was associated with male drinkers. Subjects in the present study were less negative than those tested by Jahoda and Cramond in their attitudes towards male drinkers. It has been speculated previously that the increase in positive media coverage of alcohol, particularly in the case of men, may be to some extent responsible for this shift in attitudes. In contrast, current attitudes towards smokers appear to be heading in the opposite direction, i.e. becoming more negative, especially among the younger children. Like alcohol, tobacco has become a widely publicized issue over the last twenty or so years. However, unlike much of the publicity relating to alcohol, tobacco has received a large amount of bad press, and people are now smoking much less. In view of recent data indicating a small upturn in the numbers of school-children taking up smoking, the attitudes of these younger children might, on the surface, appear more promising. However, the fact that most children of this age are similarly condemning of alcohol, the majority of whom will grow up to become drinkers themselves, suggests that such optimism should be guarded. Instead, this finding should be more realistically interpreted as a demonstration of the extent to which messages concerning tobacco have been assimilated by young children, rather that as an indication of a decline in potential smokers.

IMPLICATIONS AND RECOMMENDATIONS

The findings of this study have a number of implications for research relating to primary preventative strategies. While the majority of young people learn to consume alcohol in a reasonably sensible and safe manner, a significant minority will go on to develop problematic styles of drinking. The aetiology of problem drinking remains unclear, despite longitudinal and retrospective studies of the drinking careers of both problem and non-problem drinkers. However, data relating to individual drinking histories starting from the onset of early alcohol cognitions may eventually provide important clues in predicting the likelihood of future problems before these situations arise. This may be a long way in the future. However, there are also implications for primary preventative strategies, which could begin to be applied now.

The results of this exercise provide overwhelming evidence to support the contention that socialization to alcohol is a continuous process which begins from early childhood. In fact, the implication is that the onset of this learning occurs among children of a younger age than those studied here. While it might reasonably be argued that much of this initial knowledge is rather simplistic and often a little misguided, the crucial issue here is that young children have both the propensity and the ability to learn about alcohol.

The apparent widespread failure, at least in the short term, of most secondary-school-based alcohol education has been documented in detail in Chapter 2. As yet, it remains unclear as to which particular factors are responsible for this lack of success or, more pertinently, which elements may have contributed to the small positive achievements evident in very few cases. Underlying theories of attitudinal and behavioural change, course structures, methods of presentation, educator status, etc. have all undergone largely unsuccessful manipulations in attempts to find a successful strategy for teaching. However, one aspect which they all have in common is the group of individuals at which they are aimed – adolescents. By definition, adolescence is the final transitional stage through which children pass before attaining adulthood. It is during this time that young people tend to adopt more adult-like behaviours, including, for many, the onset of significant involvement with alcohol. Thus for these individuals the educational messages they are receiving with regard to alcohol will often be overtaken in precedence by their own personal experiences, a factor which has been highlighted by adolescents themselves (Loretto and May, 1993). It is beyond the scope of this study to state categorically the course which future alcohol education should run. However, the present findings do provide a useful basis for speculation about alternative strategies.

In the first instance, the finding that young children are both interested in and amenable to messages about alcohol, well before their own personal involvement becomes a greater issue for them, might usefully be exploited. It is true that the information young children possess with regard to alcohol is rather one-sided and simplistic. That alcohol is bad for people's health, it makes people drunk and drunks are people to be avoided, are typical statements made by these children. So ingrained do these negative ideas about alcohol become, it would appear that children are often reluctant to admit the possibility that they too will become drinkers. This evidently unrealistic expectation with regard to the majority of these children may in some way be responsible for the secretive, almost guilty way in which some adolescents first come to gain significant experience of alcohol. However, the blame for these often incorrect beliefs about alcohol should not be placed entirely on the children themselves. The results of the tasks, such as those dealing with the categorization of objects, normative perceptions and attitudes towards adult behaviour, suggest that young children do have the capacity for assimilating relevant and more accurate information about issues other than alcohol.

What is probably of more relevance here is the confounding influence of society's contradictory messages concerning alcohol. The dissemination of messages about alcohol consumption are typically highly erratic. On the one hand, there is the ubiquitous media portrayal of the normality and positive sociability of drinking, lent added credence by the fact that the vast majority of adults do themselves drink. On the other, there are the health warnings implicit and explicit within the aims of alcohol education, which are at least verbally reinforced by significant authority figures such as teachers and parents. The issue of this double standard is a pertinent one. As with a number of other countries, Britain has a rather ambivalent attitude towards alcohol; whereas, in other European regions drinking is often more likely to be perceived in a less directive light. Moreover, children in these latter areas are openly taught from an early age to view alcohol in this way, whereas in Britain, the licensing laws, or more pertinently the actions of many adults, are such that they reinforce the notion that alcohol consumption is the mysterious preserve of adults alone. This view also appears to have been reinforced throughout the United States, where the legal age of alcohol consumption or purchase has recently been raised to twenty-one years. However, in recognition of the situation in Britain, a recent Home Office report has recommended the introduction of alcohol-serving 'café-style' premises, for the use of families as opposed to adults only (1993). It is hoped that these will encourage and enable parents to introduce children to alcohol in a trouble-free and appropriate setting, as a strategy for demystifying the whole issue of alcohol consumption and weakening the association between alcohol consumption and adulthood. This would seem to be a step in the right direction, and in itself would provide a more consistent basis from which to direct future education initiatives. Of the comparable work which has been conducted, the majority has been restricted to the United States and, to a lesser extent, New Zealand. While these studies provide invaluable comparative data, the context in which drinking occurs in these countries is more similar to that in Britain than, for example, the southern Mediterranean countries. It would be extremely interesting and informative were similar studies to be carried out in these latter areas, where alcohol consumption has come to have a different symbolic or cultural value.

In addition, a more thorough appreciation of both how children come to learn about alcohol and the content of this learning is also essential if education for this age group is to be a viable alternative. In other words, educators must be sensitive to the appropriateness of educational content at different stages in the cognitive and social growth of children. Thus it should be recommended that alcohol education be a gradual and continuous process, building from an early base of knowledge and progressively developing in accordance with the development of the child. Evidently further research will be required before this can be fully realized. For, while the results reported in this book provide useful indicators relating to the early development of alcohol awareness, as yet there has been no attempt to examine this age group on a nationally representative basis.

So far, little mention has been made of the educators themselves. With regard to adolescent-based initiatives it has invariably fallen to the school to provide formalized alcohol education. However, in an age in which instruction about safe sex and illegal drug use has understandably come to the fore in light of the very immediate and potentially devastating threat of HIV/AIDS, alcohol misuse might be viewed as being less of a priority for an already overstretched system. Moreover, some teachers are beginning to express concerns about their abilities to cope with such demands (Plant, 1992), in terms of both time and personal ability. Surprisingly, little research has been directed at how teachers themselves view this issue. This is a situation which evidently needs to be rectified.

In relation to the above, another important point highlighted by the results of this study is the crucial role of the parents in the development of children's early alcohol cognitions. Familial influences on adolescent use of alcohol have also been examined in previous studies, yet current alcohol education strategies have so far failed to take into account the implications of these factors. A recent survey of student teachers has indicated that they are highly sensitive to this issue (Plant, 1992). The transmission of mixed, possibly contradictory, messages relating to alcohol from family and school can only confuse the learning process. Therefore, a concerted effort by educationalists to combine these sources might make for a more productive strategy. Research is currently being conducted on parents of young children in an attempt to discover their views, with the aim of designing a suitable package for parents to assist them when tackling this subject with their children (Fossey and Miller, 1994). For as with teachers, it cannot simply be assumed that parents will feel sufficiently equipped to deal with this type of instruction. Preliminary discussions with parents have yielded some extremely interesting information. Many are unaware of the alcohol-education policy of their children's school and strongly feel that this is a topic about which they should be informed. In addition, the majority feel that parents themselves have the ultimate responsibility for teaching their children about alcohol, and often view the role of the school as providing secondary reinforcement. These initial findings strongly highlight the need for parents and teachers to come together and discuss the possibility of joint strategies. Unfortunately, there is inevitably the risk that those families who may benefit the most from such help are less likely to participate in initiatives of this kind. Also inevitable is the fact that there will be those those who strongly disapprove of any type of alcohol education for their children, as a result, for example, of religious mores. Future research would benefit greatly by gaining access to these special groups in order that such views can also be taken into account.

In conclusion, it is clear that there is much work still needed in this area. A variety of implications and recommendations for future research, policy and education initiatives have been highlighted by the findings of this study. Ideally, what is required now is that individuals in all three areas combine resources in a concerted attempt to find workable solutions for preventative strategy.

Appendix 1

Photographs used in the 'Judgement of Photographs' task

Each subject was required to judge two sets of photographs, each set consisting of twenty-four photographs (twenty plus four repeats). Each person appeared in one set engaged in one alcohol-related activity, and in the other set in a non-alcohol-related activity or a tobacco-related activity. These activities were more or less identical to those used by Jahoda and Cramond (with the exception of the item 'playing a guitar', which replaced the original item 'playing a trumpet'). They are shown in Table A.1.

Table A.1 Activities in photographs

a	playing cards	h	drinking beer
b	playing a guitar	i	smoking a pipe
c	eating an apple	j	smoking a cigarette
d	drinking from a 'short' glass	k	reading a book
e	reading a newspaper	l	eating a cake
f	drinking milk	m	brushing hair
g	eating with a knife and fork	n	telephoning

The activities of each person in each of the two sessions are shown in Table A.2, indicating which of the photographs were repeated in order to provide consistency checks. Again, the format was the same as that employed by Jahoda and Cramond. Finally, Table A.3 shows the three random orders of presentation of the photographs for each set of photographs used in the two sessions.

Table A.2 Repeated photographs

Person No.	Activity	SET 1			Activity	SET 2		
		Repeat A	Repeat B	Repeat C		Repeat A	Repeat B	Repeat C
1	k		*	*	f		*	
2	h				n			
3	d				l			*
4	j				m	*	*	
5	l	*			j			
6	m		*		n			
7	n				d			
8	n				h			
9	f	*		*	j			
10	d				k	*		*
11	a		*		c		*	
12	b			*	i			
13	c			*	b			*
14	d				f	*		
15	e	*			d			
16	f		*		j			
17	g	*			h			
18	h				a		*	
19	i				d			
20	j				g	*		*

Persons numbered 1–10 are female; persons numbered 11–20 are male.

Table A.3 Random orders of presentation in Sessions 1 and 2

Order of presentation	SET 1			SET 2		
	A	B	C	A	B	C
1	16f	1k	13c	1f	4m	3l
2	5l	15e	7n	20g	18a	13b
3	20j	6m	4j	16j	11c	5j
4	17g	2h	12b	10k	17d	17h
5	18h	16f	1k	15d	112i	2n
6	4j	7n	14d	13b	1f	20g
7	13c	20j	5l	4m	2n	10k
8	9f	13c	19i	14f	16j	15d
9	3d	10d	15e	17h	17h	9j
10	15e	9f	3d	5j	10k	6n
11	19i	18h	9f	2n	18a*	14f
12	7n	1k*	12b*	18a	13b	16j
13	11a	11a	2h	7d	5j	7d
14	14d	12b	13c*	4m*	15d	1f
15	6m	5l	17g	12i	6n	18a
16	2h	6m*	6m	14f*	3l	12i
17	1k	14d	16f	8h	8h	4m
18	15e*	16f*	10d	3l	14f	8h
19	17g*	4j	11a	11c	4m*	11c
20	8n	8n	20j	9j	19d	10k*
21	10d	3d	8n	19d	9j	19d
22	9f*	19i	18h	6n	20g	3l*
23	5l*	17g	9f*	20g*	11c*	13b*
24	12b	11a*	1k*	10k*	1f*	20g*

* Repeated photographs.

Appendix 2

Activities used in the 'Perceived Likes and Dislikes' task

Each subject was presented with a selection of activities from either List A or List B in Session 1, and a different selection of activities from the same list in Session 2. The two lists of activities are shown in Table A.4.

The two random orders of presentation for both activity lists over both sessions are shown in Table A.5. As before, these are similar to those generated by Jahoda and Cramond.

Table A.4 Lists of activities

Activity	LIST A	LIST B
a	doing the cooking	eating chocolate[†]
b	going to school*	going to the zoo
c	digging the garden*	going to the shops*
d	eating carrots	drinking tea
e	smoking a cigarette	going to a football match
f	being punished	eating cabbage*
g	playing with marbles	playing with guns
h	drinking coffee*	doing the cooking
i	painting the house	mending a bike*
j	being nicely dressed[†]	being punished[†]
k	knitting[†]	drinking milk*
l	eating ice-cream*	being surprised
m	going to work	playing at skipping
n	drinking orange juice	taking medicine
o	mending a car	eating fish
p	playing with dolls	being nicely dressed
q	eating stew	digging the garden
r	being surprised	smoking a pipe
s	sewing on buttons[‡]	going to church
t	drinking milk	washing up dishes[‡]
u	drinking beer[†]	drinking beer[†]
v	drinking whisky[†]	drinking whisky[†]
w	going to the pub	going to the pub
x	being drunk	being drunk

* These items were repeated in Session 1.
[†] These items were repeated in Session 2.
[‡] In Session 2 these items were replaced by the item 'drinking wine'.

Table A.5 Orders of presentation of the activity lists

	Session 1				Session 2			
	List A		List B		List A		List B	
	Order (1)	Order (2)	Order (1)	Order (2)	Order (1)	Order (2)	Order (1)	Order (2)
	a	b	a	t	b	a	a	d
	b	i	b	o	k	p	j	m
	c	h	c	s	q	j	d	w
	d	j	d	d	u	w	x	q
	e	l	e	g	r	h	c	a
	f	s	f	l	o	c	i	j
	g	t	g	f	l	f	u	v
	h	k	h	h	v	v	g	i
	i	d	i	j	j	k	t	c
	j	f	j	c	g	o	e	x
	k	c	k	k	w	u	v	f
	l	b*	c*	i*	e	g	f	e
	m	n	l	r	a	e	q	t
	n	a	m	f*	c	x	j*	u
	o	q	i*	m	f	q	w	j*
	p	m	n	p	u*	s	k	a*
	q	p	o	b	h	j*	b	k
	r	c*	p	e	s	v*	v*	u*
	c*	h*	q	n	x	t	r	b
	h*	r	r	c*	p	b	p	p
	b*	e	s	k*	j*	r	n	g
	l*	l*	t	q	v*	u*	u*	v*
	s	o	f*	l	k*	k*	a*	r
	t	g	k*	a	t	l	m	n

* Repeated items in each list.

Appendix 3
Subjects' knowledge of alcohol

In order to ascertain which factors, if any, were likely to emerge as predictors of subjects' knowledge of alcohol, stepwise loglinear regression was carried out on these data, using GLIM. The findings are discussed in greater detail in the text, however, age, cognitive ability and city of subjects were all found to be significant predictors of the type of knowledge children possessed in relation to alcohol. The results of this analysis are detailed in Table A.6.

Table A.6 Predictors of subjects' knowledge of alcohol

Parameter (reference categories in brackets)	Log odds	95% C.I. ↓	↑
BPVS (high score)			
BPVS (2) low score	0.8023	0.1913	1.4115
Knowledge of alc. (nothing)			
Knowledge of alcohol (negative)	−0.4067	−1.4463	0.6329
Knowledge of alcohol (factual)	0.6214	−0.2466	1.4894
City (Edinburgh)			
City (2) Birmingham	0.2713	−0.5159	1.0585
Age (5–6 yrs)			
Age (2) 7–8 yrs	−0.3365	−1.1645	0.4915
Age (3) 9–10 yrs	−0.5596	−1.4458	0.3266
*BPVS * knowledge of alc.*			
BPVS (2) * knowledge (2)	−0.4475	−1.1825	0.2875
BPVS (2) * knowledge (3)	−1.1100	−1.8036	−0.4164
*BPVS * city*			
BPVS (2) * city (2)	0.4210	−0.1464	0.9884
*Knowledge * city*			
Knowledge (2) * city (2)	−0.5395	−1.8029	0.7239
Knowledge (3) * city (2)	−1.0310	−2.1512	0.0892
*Knowledge * age*			
Knowledge (2) * age (2)	0.7885	−0.4845	2.0165
Knowledge (2) * age (3)	0.8109	−0.5313	2.1531
Knowledge (3) * age (2)	0.5306	−0.5680	1.6292
Knowledge (3) * age (3)	0.9651	−0.1581	2.0883
*City * age*			
City (2) * age (2)	−0.3175	−1.3915	0.7565
City (2) * age (3)	−1.9660	−3.6820	−0.2500
*Knowledge * city * age*			
Knowledge (2) * city (2) * age (2)	0.5586	−1.1576	2.2748
Knowledge (2) * city (2) * age (3)	2.0940	0.7340	5.0740
Knowledge (3) * city (2) * age (2)	0.6088	−0.9666	2.1842
Knowledge (3) * city (2) * age (3)	2.0460	−0.0100	4.1020

Appendix 4
Subjects' knowledge of drunks

As with subjects' knowledge of alcohol, knowledge of drunks was analysed in order to discover any predictor variables which were likely to account for the type of knowledge subjects possessed. Stepwise loglinear regression was conducted on the data, the results of which are shown in Table A.7. As before, the findings are discussed at greater length in the text; however, age, city and cognitive ability of subjects again emerged as the only significant predictors of performance.

Table A.7 Predictors of subjects' knowledge of drunks

Parameter (reference) categories in brackets)	Log odds	95% C.I. ↓	↑
Knowledge of drunks (nothing)			
Knowledge of drunks (negative)	−0.8169	−1.5967	−0.0371
Knowledge of drunks (factual)	−0.5294	−1.3396	0.2808
City (Edinburgh)			
City (2) Birmingham	0.1135	−0.4493	0.6763
BPVS (high score)			
BPVS (2) low score	0.3320	−0.2198	0.8838
Age (5–6 yrs)			
Age (2) 7–8 yrs	−0.3536	−0.8078	0.1006
Age (3) 9–10 yrs	−1.4520	−2.1218	−0.7822
*Knowledge * city*			
Knowledge (2) * city (2)	−0.7716	−1.3766	−0.1666
Knowledge (3) * city (2)	−0.3511	−1.1079	0.4057
*Knowledge * BPVS*			
Knowledge (2) * BPVS (2)	0.0121	−0.6188	0.6429
Knowledge (3) * BPVS (2)	−0.8873	−1.6473	−0.1273
*City * BPVS*			
City (2) * BPVS (2)	0.5514	−0.0118	1.1146
*Knowledge * age*			
Knowledge (2) * age (2)	1.0470	0.2502	1.8438
Knowledge (2) * age (3)	2.7640	1.8632	3.6648
Knowledge (3) * age (2)	0.5478	−0.3050	1.4006
Knowledge (3) * age (3)	1.3780	0.3572	2.3988

Bibliography

Adair, J.G. (1984) 'The Hawthorne effect: a reconsideration of the methodological artefact', *Journal of Applied Psychology*, 69: 344–5.

Ahlstrom, S. (1987) 'Young people's drinking habits', in J. Simpura (ed.) *Finnish Drinking Habits*, Finnish Foundation for Alcohol Studies.

—— (1988) 'A comparative study of adolescent drinking habits', paper presented at the First Annual Meeting of the Kettil Bruun Society, Berkeley, CA, June.

Ahlstrom-Laasko, S. (1975) 'Changing drinking habits among Finnish youth', report from the Social Research Institute of Alcohol Studies, no. 81, Helsinki.

Aitken, P.P. (1978) 'Ten-to-fourteen year-olds and alcohol', Edinburgh: HMSO.

Aitken, P.P. and Jahoda, G. (1983) 'An observational study of young adults' drinking groups I: drink preferences, demographic and structural variables as predictors of alcohol consumption', *Alcohol & Alcoholism*, 18(2): 135–50.

—— (1985) 'An observational study of young adults' drinking groups II: drink purchasing procedures, group pressures and alcohol consumption by companions as predictors of alcohol consumption', *Alcohol and Alcoholism*, 20: 445–57.

Aitken, P.P. and Leathar, D.S. (1981) 'Adults' attitudes towards drinking and smoking among young people in Scotland', Edinburgh: HMSO.

Aitken, P.P., Eadie, D.R., Leathar, D.S., McNeill, R.E.J. and Scott, A.C. (1988) 'Television advertisements for alcoholic drinks do reinforce underage drinking', *British Journal of Addiction*, 83: 1399–1419.

Aitken P.P., Leathar, D.S., Scott, A.C. (1988) 'Ten-to sixteen year-olds' perceptions of advertisements for alcoholic drinks', *Alcohol and Alcoholism*, 23(6): 491–500.

Akers, R.L. (1985) *Deviant Behaviour: A Social Learning Approach*, Belmont, CA: Wadsworth.

Amos, A. and Hillhouse, A. (1992) *Tobacco Use in Scotland: A Review of Literature and Research*, Edinburgh: ASH.

Armyr, G. (1985) 'Trends in abstinence and alcohol consumption among youth in Sweden', paper presented at the ICAA meeting, Rome, June.

Atkin, C., Hocking, J. and Block, M. (1984) 'Teenage drinking: does advertising make a difference?', *Journal of Communication*, 34: 157–67.

Atkin, C.K., Neuendorf, K. and McDermott, S. (1983) 'The role of alcohol advertising in excessive and hazardous drinking', *Journal of Drug Education*, 13: 313–25.

Bagnall, G.M. (1988) 'Use of alcohol, tobacco and illicit drugs amongst 13-year-olds in three areas of Britain', *Drug and Alcohol Dependence*, 22: 241–51.

—— (1991) *Educating Young Drinkers*, London: Routledge.

Bandura, A. (1977) *Social Learning Theory*, Englewood Cliffs, NJ: Prentice-Hall.

—— (1986) *The Social Foundations of Thought and Action: A Social Cognitive Theory*, Englewood Cliffs, NJ: Prentice-Hall.

Bangert-Drowns, R.L. (1988) 'The effects of school-based substance abuse education – a meta-analysis', *Journal of Drug Education*, 18: 243–64.

Barnea, Z., Rahav, G. and Teichman, M. (1987) 'The reliability and consistency of self-reports on substance use in a longitudinal study', *British Journal of Addiction*, 82(8): 891–8.

Barnes, G. (1977) 'The development of adolescent drinking behaviour: an evaluative review of the impact of the socialisation process within the family', *Adolescence*, 12: 571–91.

Barnes, G., Farrell, M. and Cairns, A. (1986) 'Parental socialization factors and adolescent drinking behaviours', *Journal of Marriage and the Family*, 48: 27–36.

Bastide, H. (1954) 'Une enquête sur l'opinion publique à l'égard de l'alcoolisme', *Population*, 9: 13–42.

Berndt, T.J. and Heller, K.A. (1985) 'Measuring children's personality attributions: responses to open-ended questions versus trait ratings and predictions of future behaviour', in S.R. Yussen (ed.) *The Growth of Reflection in Children*, New York: Academic Press, 349–74.

Biddle, B.J., Bank, B.J. and Marlin, M.M. (1980) 'Social determinants of adolescent drinking', *Journal of Studies on Alcohol*, 41(3): 215–41.

Blane, H.T. (1977) 'Education and prevention of alcoholism', in B. Kissin and H. Begleiter (eds) *Biology of Alcoholism: Social Aspects of Alcoholism*, (vol. 4). New York: Plenum Press.

Bloom, B. *et al.* (1956) *Taxonomy of Educational Objectives, Cognitive Domain*, New York: David McKay.

Borgida, E., Locksley, A. and Brekke, N. (1981) 'Social stereotypes and social judgment', in N. Cantor and J.F. Kihlstrom (eds) *Personality, Cognition and Social Interaction*, Hillsdale, NJ: Erlbaum, 153–69.

Botvin, G.J. (1982) 'Broadening the focus of smoking prevention strategies', in T.J. Coates, A.C. Peterson and C. Perry (eds) *Promoting Adolescent Health: A Dialog on Research and Practice*, Orlando, FL: Academic Press, 137–48.

Botvin, G.J., Baker, E., Botvin, E.N., Filazolla, A.D. and Millmann, R.B. (1984a) 'Prevention of alcohol misuse through the development of personal and social competence: a Pilot Study', *Journal of Studies on Alcohol*, 45: 550–2.

—— (1984b) 'A cognitive-behavioural approach to substance abuse prevention', *Addictive Behaviours*, 9: 137–47.

Botvin, G.J., Baker, E., Filazolla, A.D. and Botvin, E.M. (1990) 'A cognitive-behavioural approach to substance abuse prevention: one-year follow-up', *Addictive Behaviours*, 15: 47–63.

Braucht, G.N. and Braucht, B. (1984) 'Prevention of problem drinking among youth: evaluation of educational strategies', in P.M. Miller and T.D. Nirenberg (eds) *Prevention of Alcohol Abuse*, New York: Plenum Press.

Breed, W. and DeFoe, J.R. (1978) 'Drinking on television: a comparison of alcohol use to the use of coffee, tea, soft drinks, water and cigarettes', *The Bottom Line*, 2(1): 28–9.

—— (1981) 'The portrayal of the drinking process on prime-time television', *Journal of Communication*, 31: 58–67.

Brewers' Society (1992) *Statistical Handbook: A Compilation of Drinks Industry Statistics*, London: Brewing Publications Ltd.

—— (1993) *Statistical Handbook: A Compilation of Drinks Industry Statistics*, London: Brewing Publications Ltd.

Brigham, J.C. (1991) *Social Psychology*, 2nd edn, New York: HarperCollins.

British Medical Association (1986) *Young People and Alcohol*, London: British Medical Association.

Bronfenbrenner, U. (1962) 'The role of age, sex, class and culture in studies of moral development', Religious Education, 57: 3–17.

Brook, J.E. and Brook, J.S. (1988) 'A developmental approach examining social and personal correlates in relation to alcohol use over time', *Journal of General Psychology*, 149: 93–110.

Brown, S.A, Goldman, M.S, Inn, A. and Anderson, L.R. (1980) 'Expectations of reinforcement from alcohol: their domain and relation to drinking patterns', *Journal of Consulting and Clinical Psychology*, 48: 419–26.

Bruvold, W.H. and Rundall, T.G. (1985) 'A meta-evaluation of California School based adolescent smoking and alcohol use reduction programs', Sacramento, CA: Department of Health Sciences.

—— (1988) 'A meta-analysis and theoretical review of school-based tobacco and alcohol intervention programs', *Psychology and Health*, 2: 53–78.

Cafiso, J., Goodstadt, M.S., Garlington, W.K., Sheppard, M.A. (1982) 'Television portrayal of alcohol and other beverages', *Journal of Studies on Alcohol*, 43(11): 1232–43.

Cahalan, D. and Room, R. (1974) 'Problem drinking among American men', New Brunswick, NJ: Rutgers Center of Alcohol Studies, Monograph no. 7.

Cahalan, D., Cisin, I.H. and Crossley, H.M. (1969) *American Drinking Practices: A National Study of Drinking Behaviour and Attitudes*, New Brunswick, NJ: Rutgers Center of Alcohol Studies, Monograph no. 4.

Cain, W.S. (1979) 'To know with the nose: keys to odour identification', *Science*, 203: 467–70.

—— (1982) 'Odour identification by males and females: predictions vs performance', *Chemical Senses*, 7(2): 129–42.

Caleekal-John, A. and Pletsch, D.H. (1984) 'An interdisciplinary approach to alcohol education in the university curriculum', *Journal of Alcohol and Drug Education*, 30: 50–60.

Casswell, S. (1982) 'Alcohol use by Auckland high school students', *New Zealand Medical Journal*, 95: 856–8.

Casswell, S., Gilmore, L., Silva, P. and Brasch, P. (1983) 'Early experiences with alcohol: a survey of an eight and nine year old sample', *New Zealand Medical Journal*, 96: 1001–3.

Casswell, S., Brasch, P., Gilmore, L. and Silva, P. (1985) 'Children's attitudes to alcohol and awareness of alcohol-related problems', *British Journal of Addiction*, 80(2): 191–4.

Casswell, S., Gilmore, L., Silva, P. and Brasch, P. (1988) 'What children know about alcohol and how they know it', *British Journal of Addiction*, 83: 223–7.

Central Statistical Office (1992) *Regional Trends 27*, London: HMSO.

—— (1993) *Social Trends 23*, London: HMSO.

Charlton, A. (1984) 'Children's opinions about smoking', *Journal of the Royal College of General Practitioners*, 34: 483–7.

Charlton, A. and Blair, V. (1989) 'Predicting the onset of smoking in boys and girls', *Social Science and Medicine*, 29: 813–8.

Chassin, L., Presson, C.C., Sherman, S.J. and McGrew, J. (1987) 'The changing smoking environment for middle and high school students: 1980–1983', *Journal of Behavioural Medicine*, 10: 581–93.

Christiansen, B.A., Goldman, M.S. and Inn, A. (1982) 'Development of alcohol-related expectancies in adolescents: separating pharmacological from social-learning influences', *Journal of Consulting & Clinical Psychology*, 50(3): 336–44.

Clark, E.V. (1983) 'Meaning and concepts', in P.H. Mussen *Handbook of Child Psychology*, vol. 3, J.H. Flavell and E.M. Markman (eds) *Cognitive Development*, New York: Wiley.

Clayton, R.R. and Lacey, W.B. (1982) 'Interpersonal influences on male drug use and drug use intentions', *International Journal of the Addictions*, 17: 655–66.

Cohen, S. (1972) *Folk Devils and Moral Panics*, London: Granada.

Cook, S.W. and Selltiz, C. (1964) 'A multiple indicator approach to attitude measurement', in N. Warren and M. Jahoda (eds) *Attitudes*, 2nd edn, Harmondsworth: Penguin, 364–94.

Cooke, G., Wehmer, G. and Gruber, J. (1975) 'Training paraprofessionals in the treatment of alcoholism', *Quarterly Journal of Studies on Alcohol*, 36(7): 938–48.

Coombs, R.H. and Paulson, M.J. (1988) 'Contrasting family patterns of adolescent drug users and nonusers', *Journal of Chemical Dependency Treatment*, 1: 59–72.

Corti, B., Binns, C.W., Howatt, P.A., Blaze-Temple, D. and Lo, S.K. (1990) 'Comparison of 7-day retrospective and prospective alcohol consumption in Perth, Western Australia – methodological issues', *British Journal of Addiction*, 85(3): 379–88.

Currie, C. and Todd, J. (1992) *Health Behaviours of Scottish Schoolchildren: Reports 1 and 2*, Edinburgh: HEBS/RUHBC.

Dale, E. and Reichert, D. (1957) *Bibliography of Vocabulary Studies*, Colombus, OH: Ohio State University Bureau of Educational Research.

Davies, J. and Stacey, B. (1972) *Teenagers and Alcohol: A Developmental Study in Glasgow*, London: HMSO.

De Haes, W.F.M. (1987) 'Looking for effective drug education programmes: 15 years explanation of the effects of different drug education programmes', *Health Education Research – Theory and Practice*, 2: 433–8.

DeFoe, J.R., Breed, W. and Breed, L.A. (1983) 'Drinking on television: a five-year study', *Journal of Drug Education*, 13: 25–83.

Degnan, E.J. (1972) 'An exploration into the relationship between depression and positive attitude towards drugs in young adolescents and the evaluation of a drug education program', *Dissertations Abstract*, 32 (110B): 6614–5.

Department of Transport (1990) *Road Accidents in Great Britain: The Casualty Report*, London: HMSO.

Dight, S. (1976) *Scottish Drinking Habits*, London: HMSO.

Donaldson, M. (1978) *Children's Minds*, Great Britain: Fontana.

Donaldson, M.L. and Elliot, A. (1990) 'Children's explanations', in R. Grieve and M. Hughes (eds) *Understanding Children*, Oxford: Basil Blackwell, 26–50.

Dorn, N. (1983) *Alcohol, Youth and the State: Drinking Practices, Controls and Health Education*, London: Croom Helm.

Doty, R.L., Shaman, P., Applebaum, S.L., Giberson, R., Sikorski, L., Rosenberg, L. (1984) 'Smell identification ability: changes with age', *Science*, 226: 1441–3.

Doty, R.L., Applebaum, S., Zushos, H., Settle, R.G. (1985) 'Sex differences in odour identification ability: a cross-cultural analysis', *Neuropsychologia*, 23(5): 667–72.

Duffy, J.C. and Waterton, J.J. (1984) 'Under reporting of alcohol consumption in sample surveys: the effect of computer interviewing in field work', *British Journal of Addiction*, 79(3): 303–8.

Dunn, L.M. (1959), *Peabody Picture Vocabulary Test Manual*, Circle Pines, MN: American Guidance Service.

Dunn, L.M. and Dunn, L.M. (1981) *Peabody Picture Vocabulary Test - Revised Manual*, Circle Pines, MN: American Guidance Service.

Dunn, L.M., Dunn, L.M., Whetton, C., Pintilie, D. (1982) *British Picture Vocabulary Scale*, Windsor: NFER-Nelson.

Eisler, D. (1983) *A Lifting of Liquor Ban*, Toronto: Macleans.

Elliot, C.D. (1982) *The British Ability Scales, Manual 2: Technical and Statistical Information*, Windsor: NFER-NELSON.

Engen, T. (1987) 'Remembering odours and their names', *American Scientist*, 75: 497–503.

Fagot, B.I. (1985) 'Beyond the reinforcement principle: another step towards understanding sex role development', *Developmental Psychology*, 21: 1097–104.

Fazio, R.H. and Zanna, M.P. (1981) 'Direct experience and attitude-behaviour consistency', in L. Berkowitz (ed.) *Advances in Experimental Social Psychology*, vol. 14, New York: Academic Press, 162–202.

Feldman, N.S. and Ruble, D.N. (1981) 'The development of person perception: cognitive and social factors', in S.S. Brehm, S.M. Kassin, and F.X. Gibbons, (eds) *Developmental Social Psychology: Theory and Research*, Oxford: Oxford University Press.

Fillmore, K.M. (1984) ' "When angels fall": women's drinking as a cultural preoccupation and as a reality', in S.C. Wilsnack and L.J. Beckman (eds) *Alcohol Problems in Women, Consequences and Interventions*, New York: Guildford Press, 7–36.

—— (1988) *Alcohol Use across the Life Course*, Toronto: Addiction Research Foundation.

Finn, T.A. and Strickland, D.E. (1982) 'A content analysis of beverage alcohol advertising: II television advertising', *Journal of Studies on Alcohol*, 43: 964–89.

Fisher, J., Cross, D., Carrill, T. and Murray, P. (1987) 'Alcohol consumption and young people in Australia', *Health Education Journal*, 46: 116–22.

Flay, B.R. and Sobel, J.J. (1983) 'The role of mass media in preventing adolescent substance abuse', in T.J. Glynn, C.G. Leukefeld and J.P. Ludford (eds) *Preventing Adolescent Drug Abuse: Intervention Strategies*, NIDA Research Monograph no. 47, DHHS Publication no. (ADM) 83–1280, Washington: Government Printing Office.

Ford, M.E. (1982) 'Social cognition and social competence in adolescence', *Developmental Psychology*, 18: 323–40.

Fossey E. (1992) 'Alcohol and young children', paper presented at national conference of Addictions Forum, on alcohol and young people, London, October.

Fossey, E. and Miller, P. (1994) *Parents and Alcohol Education – A Study in Three Areas*, interim report to the Portman Group, London.

Foster, K., Wilmot, A. and Dobbs, J. (1990) *General Household Survey 1988*, London: HMSO.

Foxcroft, D.R. and Lowe, G. (1991) 'Adolescent drinking behaviour and family socialisation factors: a meta-analysis' *Journal of Adolescence* 14: 255–73.

—— (1992) 'Family socialisation factors and alcohol use in older teenagers', paper presented at the 36th International Congress on Alcohol and Drug Dependence, Glasgow, Scotland, 16–21 August 1992.

Freour, P., Serise, M., Coudray, P. and Benier, J. (1969) 'Que pensent de l'alcoolisme les habitants des grands ensembles urbains?', *Revue de l'alcoolisme*, 15: 97–134.

Fritzen, R. and Mazer, G. (1975) 'The effects of fear appeals and communication upon attitudes toward alcohol consumption', *Journal of Drug Education*, 5: 171–81.

Futch, E. (1984) 'The influence of televised alcohol consumption on children's social problems solving', PhD dissertation, State University of New York.

Gaines, L.S., Maisto, S.A., Brooks, P.H., Shagena, M.M. and Dietrich, M.S. (1986) 'Development of drinking: children's knowledge of alcohol and drinking', unpublished dissertation, Department of Psychiatry, Vanderbilt University Medical School, Nashville TN.

Gaines, L.S., Brooks, P.H., Maisto, S., Dietrich, M. and Shagena, M. (1988) 'The development of children's knowledge of alcohol and the role of drinking', *Journal of Applied Developmental Psychology*, 9: 441–57.

Garbarino, J. and Bronfenbrenner, U. (1976) 'The socialisation of moral judgement and behaviour in cross-cultural perspective', in T. Lickona (ed.) *Moral Development and Behaviour: Theory, Research, and Social Issues*, New York: Holt, Rinehart and Winston, 70–83.

Gerbner, G., Morgan, M. and Signorielli, N. (1982) 'Programming health portrayals: what viewers see. say and do', in D. Pearl, L. Bouthilet and J. Lazar (eds) *Television and Behaviour: Ten Years of Scientific Progress and*

Implications for the Eighties, vol. 2, DHHS Publication no. (ADM) 82–1196, Washington: Government Printing Office, 291–307.

Gerbner, G., Gross, M., Morgan, M. and Signorielli, N. (1986), 'Living with television: the dynamics of the cultivation process', in J. Bryant and D. Zillman (eds) *Perspectives on Media Effects*, Hillsdale, NJ: Lawrence Erlbaum.

Ghodsian, M. and Power, C. (1987) 'Alcohol consumption between the ages of 16 and 23 in Britain: a longitudinal study', *British Journal of Addiction*, 82(2): 175–80.

Gillies, P. and Wilcox, B. (1984) 'Reducing the risk of smoking amongst the young', *Public Health*, 98: 49–54.

Glassner, B. and Laughlin, J. (1987) Drugs in Adolescent Worlds, London: MacMillan Press.

Globetti, G. and Harrison, D.E. (1970) 'Attitudes of high school students towards alcohol education', *Journal of School Health*, 40: 36–9.

Glynn, T. (1981) 'From family to peers: a review of transitions in influence among drug using youth', *Journal of Youth and Adolescence*, 10: 363–83.

Goddard, E. (1989) *Smoking Among Secondary School Children in England in 1988*, London: HMSO.

—— (1990) *Why Children Start Smoking*, London: HMSO.

—— (1991) *Drinking in England and Wales in the late 1980s*, London: HMSO.

Goddard, E. and Ikin, C. (1988) *Drinking in England and Wales in 1987*, London: HMSO.

Goodman, J.F. (1990) 'Variations in children's conceptualisations of mental retardation as a function of inquiry methods', *Journal of Child Psychology and Psychiatry*, 31: 935–48.

Goodstadt, M.S. (1981) 'Planning and evaluation of alcohol education programmes', *Journal of Alcohol & Drug Education*, 26(2): 1–10.

—— (1985) 'Shaping drinking practices through education', in J.P. van Wartburg, P. Magnenat, R. Müller and S. Wyss (eds) *Currents in Alcohol Research and the Prevention of Alcohol Problems*, Toronto: Hans Huber, 85–106.

Goodstadt, M.S. and Sheppard, M.A. (1983) 'Three approaches to alcohol education', *Journal of Studies on Alcohol*, 44: 362–80.

Governali, J. and Sechrist, W. (1980) 'Clarifying values in a health education setting: an experimental analysis', *Journal of School Health*, 50: 151–4.

Graham, K. (1993) 'Bars and violence', paper presented at the Addictions Forum meeting, 'Safer Bars? Safer Streets?', London, April.

Grant, M. (1982) 'Young people and alcohol problems: educating for individual and social change', paper presented at the 10th International Congress of the International Association for Child and Adolescent Psychiatry and Allied Professions, 25–30 July.

Green, L. (1979) 'National policy in the promotion of health', *International Journal of Health Education*, 22: 161–8.

Greenberg, B.S, Fernandez-Collado, C., Graef, D., Korzenny, F. and Atkin, C.K. (1979) 'Trends in use of alcohol and other substances on television', *Journal of Drug Education*, 9: 243–53.

Greenberg, G.S., Zucker, R.A. and Noll, R.B. (1985) 'The development of cognitive structures about alcoholic beverages among preschoolers', paper presented at the annual meeting of the American Psychological Association, LA, California, August.

Greenberg, M., Siegal, J. and Leitch, C. (1983) 'The nature and importance of attachment relationships to parents and to peers during adolescence', *Journal of Youth and Adolescence*, 12: 373–83.

Gunter, B. and McAleer, J.L. (1990) *Children and Television: The One-Eyed Monster?*, London: Routledge.

Hansen, A. (1985) 'Will the Government's mass media campaign on drugs work?' *British Medical Journal*, 290: 1054–55.

Hansen, W.B. (1992) 'School-based substance abuse prevention: a review of the state of the art in curriculum, 1980–1990', *Health and Education Research*, 7: 403–30.

Hansen, W.B., Johnson, C.A., Flay, B.R., Graham, J.W. and Sobel, J. (1988) 'Affective and social influences to the prevention of multiple substance abuse among 7th grade students: results from project SMART', *Preventive Medicine* 17: 135–54.

Hanson, D.J. (1980) 'Drug education: does it work?' in F.R. Sarpitti and S.K. Datesman (eds), *Drugs and the Youth Culture*, Beverley Hills, California: Sage Publications.

Harford, T.C. (1983) 'A contextual analysis of drinking events', *International Journal of the Addictions*, 18: 825–34.

Harford, T.C. and Grant, B.F. (1987) 'Psychosocial factors in adolescent drinking contexts', *Journal of Studies on Alcohol*, 48: 551–7.

Harford, T.C. and Spiegler, D.L. (1983) 'Developmental trends of adolescent drinking', *Journal of Studies on Alcohol*, 44: 181–8.

Hauge, R. and Nordlie, O. (1983) 'Paliteligheten av selvrapportert stoffbruk blant ungdom', *Nordisk tidsskrift for Kriminalvidenskab*, 70: 145–58.

Hawker, A. (1978) *Adolescents and Alcohol*, London: B. Edsall.

Haworth, A. (1985) 'Youth and alcohol in Zambia', paper prepared for the International Symposium on the Extent and Nature of Adolescent Alcohol Use, Washington, 29 July–2 August.

Health Education Authority (1989) *Teenage Health and Lifestyles*, vol. 2: *Alcohol*, London: HMSO.

—— (1990) *Young Adults' Health and Lifestyles: Alcohol*, London: MORI.

Hibell, B. (1981) 'Trends in drinking and drug habits in Swedish youth from 1971 to 1980', paper presented at the 27th International Institute on the Prevention and Treatment of Alcoholism, Vienna.

—— (1985) 'Adolescent drinking and drinking problems in Sweden', paper presented at the International Symposium on the Extent and Nature of Adolescent Alcohol Use, Washington, July.

Higgins, E.T. (1981) 'Role-taking and social judgement', in J.H. Flavell and L. Ross (eds) *Social Cognitive Development: Frontiers and Possible Futures*, New York: Cambridge University Press, 119–53.

Higgins, E.T., Feldman, N.S. and Ruble, D.N. (1980) 'Accuracy and differentiation in social prediction: a developmental perspective', *Journal of Personality*, 48(4): 520–40.

Higgins, E.T., Ruble, D.N. and Hartup, W.W. (1983) *Social Cognition and Social Development*, New York: Cambridge University Press.

Higgins, T.E. and Parsons, J.E. (1983) 'Social cognition and the social life of the child: stages and subcultures', in T.E. Higgins, D.N. Ruble, and W.W.

Hartup (eds) *Social Cognition and Social Development: A Socio-Cultural Perspective*, New York: Cambridge University Press.

Home Office (1985) *Tackling Drug Misuse: A Summary of the Government's Strategy*, London: HMSO.

—— (1993) *Possible Reforms of the Liquor Licensing System in England and Wales: A Consultation Paper*, London: Home Office.

Home Office Statistical Bulletin (1992) *Offences of Drunkenness: England and Wales 1990*, London: Home Office.

Horowitz, E.L. (1947) 'Development of attitude toward Negroes', in T.M. Newcomb and E.L. Hartley (eds) *Readings in Social Psychology*, New York: Henry Holt, 505–17..

Horton, D. (1991) 'Alcohol use in primitive societies', in D.J. Pittman and H.R. White (eds) *Society, Culture and Drinking Patterns Reexamined*, New Brunswick NJ: Rutgers Centre of Alcohol Studies.

Huba, G.J., Wingard, J.A. and Bentler, P.M. (1980) 'Applications of a theory of drug use to prevention programs', *Journal of Drug Education*, 10: 25–38.

Hughes, M. and Grieve, R. 'Interpretation of bizarre questions in five- and seven-year-old children', (in preparation).

Inhelder, B. and Piaget, J. (1964) *The Early Growth of Logic in the Child: Classification and Seriation*, London: Routledge & Kegan Paul.

Jacobsen, M., Atkins, R. and Hacker, G. (1983) *The Booze Merchants: The Inebriating of America*, Washington DC: Center for Science in the Public Interest.

Jahoda, G. and Cramond, J. (1972) *Children and Alcohol*, London: HMSO.

Jahoda, G,, Davies, J.B. and Tagg, S. (1980) 'Parents' alcohol consumption and children's knowledge of drinks and usage patterns', *British Journal of Addiction*, 75(3): 297–303.

Jessor, R. (1982) 'Critical issues in research on adolescent health promotion', in T. Coates, A. Peterson and C. Perry, (eds) *Promoting Adolescent Health*, New York: Academic Press.

Jessor, R. and Jessor, S.L. (1978) 'Theory testing in longitudinal research on marihuana use', in D.B. Kandel (ed.) *Longitudinal Research on Drug Use*, New York: Halstead Press.

Johnston, G.M,, Schantz, F.C. and Locke, T.P. (1984) 'Relationships between adolescent drug use and parental drug behaviours', *Adolescence*, 19: 295–9.

Kandel, D.B. (1982) 'Epidemiological and psychosocial perspectives on adolescent drug use', *Journal of the American Academy of Child Psychiatry*, 21: 328–47.

Kandel, D. and Lesser, G. (1972) *Youth in Two Worlds*, San Francisco: Jossey-Bass.

Kandel, D., Kessler, R.C. and Margulies, R.S. (1978) 'Antecedents of adolescent initiation into stages of drug use: a developmental analysis', in D. Kandel (ed.) *Longitudinal Research in Drug Use: Empirical Findings and Methodological Issues*, Washington, DC: Hemisphere-Wiley, 73–99.

Katz, D. (1960) 'The functional approach to the study of attitudes', *Public Opinion Quarterly*, 24: 163–204.

Katz, D. and Stotland, E. (1959) 'A preliminary statement to a theory of attitude structure and change', in S. Kock (ed.) *Psychology: A Study of a Science*, vol. 3, New York: McGraw-Hill, 423–75.

Keil, F.C. (1983) 'Semantic inferences and the acquisition of word meaning', in T.B. Seiler and W. Wannemacher (eds) *Concept Development and the Development of Word Meaning*, Berlin: Springer-Verlag.

Kelman, H.C. (1958) 'Compliance, identification and internalization', *Journal of Conflict Resolution*, 2: 51–60.

Kinder, B.N., Pape, N.E. and Walfish, S. (1980) 'Drug and alcohol education programmes: a review of outcome studies', *International Journal of the Addictions* 15: 1035–54.

Kissin, B. (1974) 'The pharmacodynamics and natural history of alcoholism', in B. Kissin and H. Begleiter (eds) *The Biology of Alcoholism*, vol. 3, New York: Plenum.

Koelega, H.S. and Köster, E. P. (1974) 'Some experiments on sex differences in odour perception', *Annals of the New York Academy of Science*, 237: 235–46.

Kohlberg, L. (1969) 'Stage and sequence: the cognitive-developmental approach to socialization', in D.A. Goslin (ed.) *Handbook of Socialization Theory and Research*, Chicago: Rand McNally, 347–480.

Kotch, J.B., Coulter, M.L., Lipsitz, A. (1986) 'Does television drinking influence children's attitudes toward alcohol?', *Addictive Behaviours*, 11: 67–70.

Lader, D. and Matheson, J. (1991) *Smoking among Secondary School Children in 1990*, London: HMSO.

Landrine, H., Bardwell, S. and Dean, T. (1988) 'Gender expectations for alcohol use: a study of the significance of masculine role', *Sex Roles*, 19: 703–12.

Lang, A.R., Winiarski, M.G. and Curtin, L. (1992) 'Person perception as a function of drinking behaviour, gender and sex role stereotypes', *Journal of Studies on Alcohol*, 53(3): 225–32.

Lawless, H.T. and Engen, T. (1977) 'Association to odours: interference, memories and verbal labelling', *Journal of Experimental Psychology*, 3: 52–9.

Leming, J.S. (1980–1) 'Curricular effectiveness in moral/values education: a review of research', *Journal of Moral Education*, 10: 147–64.

Lemmens, P., Knibbe, R.A., Tan, F. (1988) 'Weekly recall and diary estimates of alcohol consumption in a general population survey', *Journal of Studies on Alcohol*, 49: 131–5.

Livesley, W.J. and Bromley, D.B. (1973) *Person Perception in Childhood and Adolescence*, London: John Wiley, 16–31.

Loretto, W. (1993a) 'Youthful drinking in Northern Ireland and Scotland: results from a comparative study', paper presented at annual meeting of the Kettil Bruun Society, Krakow, Poland, June.

Loretto, W. and May, C. (1993) *Periodic Heavy Drinking: A Qualitative Study of Key Sub-Groups*, Report to Health Education Board for Scotland.

MacAndrew, C. and Edgerton, R.B. (1969) *Drunken Comportment: A Social Explanation*, Chicago: Aldine.

Maccoby, E.E. and Jacklin, C.N. (1974) *The Psychology of Sex Differences*, Stanford CA: Stanford University Press.

McGuire, W. (1974) 'Communication – persuasion models for drug education', in M. Goodstadt (ed.) *Research on Methods and Programs of Drug Education*, Toronto: Addiction Research Foundation.

—— (1976) 'Attitude change and the information-processing paradigm', in E. Hollander and R. Hunt (eds) *Current Perspectives in Social Psychology*, New York: Oxford University Press.

McKechnie, R.J., Cameron, D., Cameron, I.A. and Drewery, J. (1977) 'Teenage drinking in South West Scotland', *British Journal of Addiction*, 72(3): 287–95.

Maddox, G.L. (1970) *The Domesticated Drug: Drinking Among Collegians*, New Haven: College and University Press.

Makela, K. (1984) 'Permissible starting age for drinking in four Scandinavian countries', *Journal of Studies on Alcohol*, 45: 522–7.

Mardigal, S.E. and Miguez, L.H. (1985) 'Adolescent Drinking Patterns in Costa Rica', paper prepared for the International Symposium on the Extent and Nature of Adolescent Alcohol Use, Washington, 29 July–2 August.

Margulies, R.Z, Kessler, R.C. and Kandel, D.B. (1977) 'A longitudinal study of onset of drinking among high-school students', *Journal of Studies on Alcohol* 38: 897–912.

Markman, E.M., Cox, B., Machida, S. (1981) 'The standard object-sorting tasks as a measure of conceptual organisation', *Developmental Psychology*, 17: 115–17.

Marlatt, G.A. and Rohsenow, D. (1980), 'Cognitive process in alcohol use: expectancy and the balanced placebo design' in N.K. Mello (ed.) *Advances in Substance Abuse: Behavioural and Biological Research*, Greenwich, CT: JAI Press, 159–99.

Marsh, A., Dobbs, J. and White, A. (1986) *Adolescent Drinking*, London: HMSO.

Martin, C.L. and Halverson, C.F. Jnr (1981) 'A schematic processing model of sex typing and stereotyping in children', *Child Development*, 52: 1119–34.

—— (1983) 'The effects of sex-typing schemes on young children's memory', *Child Development*, 54: 563–74.

May, C. (1991) 'Research on alcohol education for young people: a critical review of the literature', *Health Education Journal*, 50: 195–9.

—— (1992) 'A burning issue? Adolescent alcohol use in Britain 1970–1991', *Alcohol and Alcoholism*, 27: 109–15.

Medina-Cardenas, E. (1985) 'The extent and nature of alcohol use among adolescents in Chile', paper prepared for the International Symposium on the Extent and Nature of Adolescent Alcohol Use, Washington, 29 July–2 August.

Mervis, C.B. and Mervis, C.A. (1982) 'Leopards are kitty-cats: object labelling by mothers for their 13 month olds', *Child Development*, 53: 267–73.

Midanik, L. (1982a) 'The validity of self-reported alcohol consumption and alcohol problems: a literature review', *British Journal of Addiction*, 77(3): 357–82.

—— (1982b) 'Over reports of recent alcohol consumption in a clinical population: a validity study', *Drug and Alcohol Dependence*, 9: 101–10.

Miller, P.M., Smith, G.T., Goldman, M.S. (1990) 'Emergence of alcohol expectancies in childhood: a possible critical period', *Journal of Studies on Alcohol*, 51(4): 343–9.

Millman, R.B. and Botvin, G.J. (1983) 'Substance use, misuse and abuse', in M. Levine, W.B. Carey, A.C. Crocker and R.T. Gross (eds) *Development-Behavioural Paediatrics*, New York: W.B. Saunders, 683–708.

Mischel, W. (1973) 'Toward a cognitive social learning reconceptualisation of personality', *Psychological Review*, 80: 252–83.

Mookherjee, H.N. (1984) 'Teenage drinking in rural middle Tennessee', *Journal of Alcohol and Drug Education*, 29: 49–57.

Moos, R. and Moos, B. (1986) *Family Environment Scale Test Manual*, Palo Alto, CA: Consulting Psychologists Press.

MORI (1990) *Teenage Smoking*, London: HEA.

Moskowitz, J.M. (1983) 'Preventing adolescent substance abuse through drug education', in T.J. Glynn, C.G. Leukefeld and J.P. Ludford (eds) *Preventing Adolescent Drug Abuse: Intervention Strategies*, NIDA Research Monograph 47, DHHS Publication no. (ADM) 83–1280, Washington: Government Printing Office, 233–49.

—— (1989) 'The primary prevention of alcohol problems: a critical review of the research literature', *Journal of Studies on Alcohol*, 50: 54–88.

Needle, R., McCubbin, H., Wilson, M., Reinbeck, R., Lazar, A. and Mederer, H. (1986) 'Interpersonal influences in adolescent drug use: the role of older siblings, parents and peers', *International Journal of the Addictions*, 21: 739–66.

Neisser, U. (1987) *Concepts and conceptual Development: Ecological and Intellectual Factors in Categorisation*, Cambridge: Cambridge University Press.

Nelson, K. (1974) 'Variations in children's concepts by age and category', *Child Development*, 45: 577–84.

—— (1985) 'Alcohol advertising and media portrayals', *Journal of the Institute for Socioeconomic Studies*, 10: 67–78.

Neuendorf, K.A. (1987) 'Alcohol advertising: evidence from social science', *Medical Information, Australia*, 43: 15–20.

Newcomb, M.D., Huba, G.J. and Bentler, P.M. (1983) 'Mothers' influence on the drug use of their children: confirmatory tests of direct modeling and mediational theories', *Developmental Psychology*, 19(5): 714–26.

Newcomb, M.D., Maddahian, E., Skager, R. and Bentler, P.M. (1987) 'Substance abuse and psychosocial risk factors among teenagers: associations with sex, age, ethnicity, and the type of school', *American Journal of Drug and Alcohol Abuse*, 13: 413–33.

Noll, R.B. (1983) 'Young male offspring of alcoholic fathers: early developmental differences from the MSU Vulnerability Study', unpublished doctoral dissertation, Department of Psychology, Michigan State University, East Lansing, MI.

Noll, R.B. and Zucker, R.A. (1983) 'Developmental findings from an alcoholic vulnerability study', paper presented at the annual meeting of the American Psychological Association, Anaheim, CA, August.

Noll, R.B., Zucker, R.A., Gonzales-Maurer, G., Greenberg, G.S. (1986) 'Development of cognitive structures about alcoholic beverages among preschoolers: II', paper presented at annual meeting of the American Psychological Association, Washington DC, August.

Noll, R.B., Zucker, R.A., Greenberg, G.S. (1990) 'Identification of alcohol by smell among preschoolers: evidence for early socialisation about drugs occurring in the home', *Child Development*, 61(5): 1520–7.

O'Connor, J. (1978) *The Young Drinkers*, London: Tavistock.

—— (1985) 'Adolescent drinking and drinking problems in Ireland', paper presented at the International Symposium on the Extent and Nature of Adolescent Alcohol Use, Washington, July.

Oei, T.P.S. and Burton, A. (1990) 'Attitudes toward smoking in 7- to 9-year old children', *International Journal of Addictions*, 25(1): 43–52.

Olafsdottir, H. (1985) 'Adolescent drinking in Iceland', paper presented at the International Symposium on the Extent and Nature of Adolescent Alcohol Use, Washington, July.

Orcutt, J.D. (1991) 'The social integration of beers and peers: situational contingencies in drinking and intoxication', in D.J. Pittman and H.R. White (eds) *Society, Culture, and Drinking Patterns Reexamined*, New Brunswick, NJ: Rutgers Center of Alcohol Studies.

Pandina, R.J., White, H.R. and Milgram, G.G. (1991) 'Assessing youthful drinking patterns' in D.J. Pittman and H.R. White (eds) *Society, Culture, and Drinking Patterns Reexamined*, New Brunswick, NJ, Rutgers Center of Alcohol Studies.

Payne, C. (1985) *The GLIM System, Release 3.77 Manual*, Oxford: Nag.

Penrose, G.B. (1978) 'Perceptions of five- and six-year-old children concerning cultural drinking norms', PhD dissertation, University of California, Berkeley.

Pernanen, K. (1974) 'Validity of survey data on alcohol use', in R.J. Gibbins, Y. Israel, H. Kalant, R.E. Popham, W. Schmidt and R.G. Smart (eds) *Research Advance In Alcohol and Drug Problems*, vol. 1, New York: John Wiley.

Plant, M.A. (1992) 'Survey of student teachers' attitudes to alcohol education', report to Education and Alcohol Conference, 19 March, Edinburgh.

Plant, M.A. and Foster, J. (1991) 'Teenagers and alcohol: results of a Scottish national survey', *Drug and Alcohol Dependence*, 28: 203–10.

Plant, M.A. and Plant, M.L. (1992) *The Risk-takers: Alcohol, Drugs, Sex and Youth*, London: Tavistock/Routledge.

Plant, M.A., Kreitman, N, Miller, T.I. and Duffy, J. (1977) 'Observing public drinking', *Journal of Studies on Alcohol*, 38: 867–80.

Plant, M.A., Peck, D.F. and Stuart, R. (1982) 'Self-reported drinking habits and alcohol-related consequences amongst a cohort of Scottish teenagers', *British Journal of Addiction*, 77(1): 75–90.

Plant, M.A., Peck, D.F. and Samuel, E. (1985) *Alcohol, Drugs and School-Leavers*, London: Tavistock.

Plant, M.A., Bagnall, G. and Foster, J. (1990) 'Teenage heavy drinkers: alcohol-related knowledge, beliefs, experiences, motivation and the social context of drinking', *Alcohol and Alcoholism*, 25(6): 691–8.

Plant, M.A., Bagnall, G., Foster, J. and Sales, J. (1990) 'Young people and drinking: results of an English national survey', *Alcohol and Alcoholism*, 25(6): 685–90.

Plant, M.L. (1990) *Women and Alcohol*, World Health Organisation, Copenhagen.

—— (1993) *Alcohol and Youth: An Analysis of the Literature, 1960–1975*, Washington DC: National Institute on Alcohol Abuse and Alcoholism.

Rachal, J.V., Williams, J.R., Breham, M.L., Cavanaugh, B., Moore, R.P. and Edkerman, W.C. (1975) *A National Study of Adolescent Drinking Behaviour, Attitudes and Correlates*, Springfield, VA: NIAAA.

Rachal, J.V., Guess, L., Hubbard, R., Maisto, S.A., Cavanaugh, E.R., Waddell, R. and Benrud, C. (1980) *The Nature and Extent of Adolescent Alcohol and Drug Use: The 1974 and 1978 National Sample Studies*, Research Triangle Park, NC: Research Triangle Institute.

Rajecki, D.W. (1982) *Attitudes: Themes and Advances*, Sunderland, MA: Sinaver Associates.

Rashkonen, O. and Ahlstrom, S. (1989) 'Trends in drinking habits among Finnish youth from 1973 to 1987', *British Journal of Addiction*, 84(9): 1075–83.

Rhodes, J.E. and Jason, L.E. (1988) *Preventing Substance Abuse among Young Children and Adolescents*, London: Pergamon Press.

Rholes, W.S. and Ruble, D.N. (1984) 'Children's understanding of dispositional characteristics of others', *Child Development*, 55: 550–60.

Richardson, D.W., Nader, P.R., Rochman, K.J. and Freidman, S.B. (1972) 'Attitudes of fifth grade students to illicit psychoactive drugs', *Journal of School Health*, 42: 389–91.

Robertson, J.R. and Eisenberg, J.L. (1981) *Technical Supplement to the Peabody Picture Vocabulary Test–Revised*, Circle Pines, MN: American Guidance Service.

Roizen, R. (1981) *The World Health Organisation Study of Community Responses to Alcohol-Related Problems: A Review of Cross-Cultural Findings*, Geneva: WHO, Annex 41 to Final Report, Phase 1.

Rooney, J.F. (1982) 'Perceived differences of standards for alcohol use among American youth', *Journal of Studies on Alcohol*, 43 (11): 1069–83.

Rosenberg, M. (1979) *Conceiving the Self*, New York: Basic Books.

Rosenbluth, J., Nathan, P.E. and Lawson, D.M. (1978) 'Environmental influences on drinking by college students in a college bar: behavioural observation in the natural environment', *Addictive Behaviours*, 3: 117–21.

Ruble, D.N., Balaban, T. and Cooper, J. (1981) 'Gender constancy and the effects of sex-typed televised toy commercials', *Child Development*, 52: 667–73.

Rychtarik, R.G., Fairbank, J.A., Allen, C.M., Foy, D.W. and Drabman, R.S. (1983) 'Alcohol use in television programming: effects on children's behaviour', *Addictive Behaviours*, 8: 19–22.

Samo, J.A., Tucker, J.A. and Vuchinich, R.E. (1989) 'Agreement between self-monitoring, recall and collateral observation measures of alcohol consumption in older adults', *Behavioural Assessment*, 11: 391–409.

Schab, F.R. (1991) 'Odour memory: taking stock', *Psychological Bulletin*, 109(2): 242–51.

Schaps, E., Moskowitz, J.M., Condon, J.W. and Malvin, J.H. (1982) 'A process and outcome evaluation of a drug education course', *Journal of Drug Education*, 12: 353–64.

Schlegel, R.P., Manske, S.R. and Page, A. (1984) 'A guided decision-making programme for elementary school students: a field experiment in alcohol education', in P.M. Miller and T.D. Nirenberg (eds) *Prevention of Alcohol Abuse*, New York: Plenum Press.

Schwartz, R.H., Hayden, G.F., Getson, P.R. and DiPaola, A. (1986) 'Drinking patterns and social consequences: a study of middle-class adolescents in two private pediatric practices', *Pediatrics*, 77(2): 139–43.

Shaffer, D.R. (1989) *Developmental Psychology: Childhood and Adolescence*, 2nd edn, Pacific Grove California: Brooks/Cole.

Shantz, C.U. (1983) 'Social Cognition', in J.H. Flavell and E.M. Markman (eds) *Cognitive Development*, New York: Wiley, 495–555.

Sharp, D.J. and Lowe, G. (1989) 'Adolescents and alcohol: a review of the recent British research', *Journal of Adolescence*, 12: 295–307.

Sharp, D.J., Greer, J.M. and Lowe, G. (1988) 'The "normalisation" of under-age drinking', paper presented at the annual conference of the British Psychological Society, Leeds, April.

Sigel, I.E. (1974) 'When do we know what a child knows?', *Human Development*, 17: 201–17.

Signorielli, N. (1987) 'Drinking, sex and violence on television: the cultural indicators perspective', *Journal of Drug Education*, 17: 245–60.

Single, E., Kandel, D. and Johnson, B.D. (1975) 'The reliability and validity of drug use responses in a large scale longitudinal survey', *Journal of Drug Issues*, 5: 426–43.

Skog, O-J, (1991) 'The validity of self-reported drug use', paper presented at annual meeting of the Kettil Bruun Society, Sigtuna, Sweden, June.

Smart, R.G. (1988) 'Does alcohol advertising affect overall consumption: a review of empirical studies', *Journal of Studies on Alcohol*, 49: 314–23.

Smart, R. and Fejer, D. (1974) 'The effects of high and low fear messages about drugs', *Journal of Drug Education*, 4: 225–35.

Smith, B.C. (1973) 'Values clarification in drug education: a comparative study', *Journal of Drug Education*, 3(4): 369–76.

Smith, M.B., Brunar, J.S. and White, R.W. (1956) *Opinions and Personality*, New York: Wiley.

Snortum, J.R., Kremer, L.K. and Berger, D.E. (1987) 'Alcoholic beverage preference as a public statement: self concept and social image of college drinkers', *Journal of Studies on Alcohol*, 48(3): 243–51.

Snow, W.H., Gilchrist, L.D. and Schinke, S.P. (1985) 'A critique of progress in adolescent smoking prevention', *Child and Youth Services Review*, 7: 1–19.

Sobell, L.C., Sobell, M.B., Riley, D.M., Klajner, F., Leo, G.I., Pavan, D. and Cancilla, A. (1986) 'Effects of television programming and advertising on alcohol consumption in normal drinkers', *Journal of Studies on Alcohol*, 47: 333–40.

Sobell, M.B., Bogardis, J., Schuller, R., Leo, G.I. and Sobell, L.C. (1989) 'Is self-monitoring of alcohol consumption reactive?', *Behavioural Assessment*, 11: 447–58.

Spiegler, D.L. (1983) 'Children's attitudes toward alcohol', *Journal of Studies on Alcohol*, 44: 545–52.

Stacey, B. and Davies, J. (1970) 'Drinking behaviour in childhood and adolescence: an evaluative review', *British Journal of Addiction*, 65(3): 203–12.

Strickland, D.E. (1983) 'Advertising exposure, alcohol consumption and misuse of alcohol', in M. Grant, M. Plant and A. Williams (eds) *Economics and Alcohol*, London: Croom Helm.

Strickland, D.E., Finn, T.A. and Lambert, M.D. (1982) 'A content analysis of beverage alcohol advertising: I magazine advertising', *Journal of Studies of Alcohol*, 43(7): 655–82.

Stuart, R. (1974) 'Teaching facts about drugs: pushing or preventing?' *Journal of Educational Psychology* 66: 189–201.

Sumner. D. (1962) 'On testing the sense of smell', *Lancet* 2, 895–7.

Tether, P. and Robinson, D. (1986) *Preventing Alcohol Problems: A Guide to Local Action*, London: Tavistock Publications.

Tobler, N.S. (1986) 'Meta-analysis of 143 adolescent drug prevention programs: quantitative outcome results of program participants compared to a control or comparison group', *Journal of Drug Issues*, 16: 537–67.

Urbain, E.S. and Kendall, P.C. (1980) 'Review of social-cognitive problem-solving interventions with children', *Psychological Bulletin*, 88: 109–43.

van de Goor, L.A.M. (1990) *Situational Aspects of Adolescent Drinking Behaviour*, Maastricht: Datawyse Maastricht, Ruud Lelivela.

van Iwaarden, M.J. (1985) 'Public health aspects of the marketing of alcoholic drinks', in M. Grant (ed.) *Alcohol Policies*, Copenhagen: WHO.

Vartiainen, E., Pallonen, U., McAlister, A., Koskela, K. and Puska, P. (1986) 'Four-year follow-up results of the smoking prevention program in the North Karelia youth project', *Preventative Medicine* 15: 692–8.

Vygotsky, L.S. (1962) *Thought and Language*, Cambridge, MA: MIT Press.

Wallack, L. (1981) 'Mass media campaigns: the odds against finding behaviour change', *Health Education Quarterly*, 8: 209–60.

Wallack, L., Grube, W., Madden, P.A. and Breed, W. (1990) 'Portrayals of alcohol on prime-time television', *Journal of Studies of Alcohol*, 51(5): 428–37.

Wechsler, D. (1974) *Wechsler Intelligence Scale for Children – Revised*, New York: The Psychological Corporation.

White, H.R., Bates, M.E. and Johnson, V. (1991) 'Learning to drink: families, peer and media influences', in D.J. Pittman, and H.R. White (eds) *Society, Culture, and Drinking Patterns Reexamined*, New Brunswick, NJ: Rutgers Center of Alcohol Studies.

Wilcox, B. and Gillies, P. (1981) *A Longitudinal Cohort Study of the Effectiveness of the My Body Project*, Report to the Health Eduction Council.

Wilcox, B., Gillies, P., Wilcox, J.S. and Reid, D.S. (1981) 'Do children influence their parents' smoking?', *Health Education Journal*, 40: 5–10.

Wilks, J. (1987) 'Drinking among teenagers in Australia: research findings, problems and prospects', *Australian Drug and Alcohol Review*, 6: 207–26.

Wilks, J. and Callan, V.J. (1984) 'Similarity of university students' and their parents' attitudes towards alcohol', *Journal of Studies on Alcohol*, 45: 326–33.

Wilks, J., Callan, V.J. and Austin, D.A. (1989) 'Parent, peer and personal determinants of adolescent drinking', *British Journal of Addiction*, 84(6): 619–30.

Williams, R.E., Ward, D.A. and Gray, L.N. (1985) 'The persistence of experimentally induced cognitive change: a neglected dimension in the assessment of drug prevention programs', *Journal of Drug Education*, 15: 33–42.

Wilson, P. (1980) *Drinking in England and Wales*, London: HMSO.

Yussen, S.R. and Kane, P.T. (1985) 'Children's conception of intelligence', in S.R. Yussen (ed.) *The Growth of Reflection in Children*, New York: Academic Press, 217–41.

Zucker, R.A. (1976) 'Parental influences upon drinking patterns of their children', in M. Greenblatt and M.A. Schuckit (eds) *Alcoholism Problems in Women and Children*, New York: Grune & Stratton.

Zucker, R.A. and Harford, T.C. (1983) 'National study of the demography of adolescent drinking practices in 1980', *Journal of Studies on Alcohol*, 44: 974–85.

Zucker, R.A. and Noll, R.B. (1987) 'The interaction of child and environment in the early development of drug involvement: a far-ranging review and planned very early intervention', *Drugs and Society*, 2: 57–97.

Zucker, R.A., Fitzgerald, H.E. and Noll, R.B. (1991) 'The development of cognitive schemas about drugs among preschoolers, 1, 2', paper presented at the biennial meeting of the Society for Research in Child Development, Seattle, April.

Index